MADE TO MOVE

Active Aging Benchmarks to Improve Balance, Posture, and Mobility for Seniors

JOSEPH WEGLEY, DPT
Doctor of Physical Therapy

Made to Move
Active Aging Benchmarks to Improve Balance, Posture, and Mobility
for Seniors
Joseph Wegley © 2019

Print ISBN: 978-1-7336117-2-5
eBook ISBN: 978-1-7336117-1-8

Cover and Interior Design by: Fusion Creative Works, FusionCW.com
Lead Editor: Jennifer Regner

Published by
Made to Move, PLLC

Printed in the United States of America

This project is dedicated to my loving
family. With their support, I have
the courage to take the leap and follow
my dream.

Also, I dedicate this to all people's goals of
living a long and fruitful life. May your body
carry you wherever your spirit wants to go.

CONTENTS

Disclaimer Statement

This manual is intended to help people maximize their mobility and achieve the best quality of life possible.

If you are having difficulty effectively implementing the following information, you should schedule an appointment with a licensed physical therapist. They will be able to determine where your specific limitations are and direct you accordingly. If any of the actions in this book result in pain that lingers or worsens after the activity has been stopped, or limits your ability to carry out your daily role, consult a physical therapist for direction.

If any of these activities and exercises result in pain and discomfort that leads to symptoms of dizziness, numbness or tingling in arms or legs, severe shortness of breath, chest pain, severe pain anywhere that doesn't resolve with rest or repositioning, or focal weakness (areas of weakness in a specific part of the body, such as the leg(s), feet, arm(s), or hand), or an unexplainable increase in fear or anxiety, consult a medical professional (i.e., a physician) as soon as possible. This generally may not be emergent, but absolutely needs to be evaluated sooner than later to prevent further injury.

If you have a medical condition that you are unsure may be affected by exercise, consult a medical professional (i.e., a physician) before starting the program. The information in this manual is not meant to replace sound medical advice that is specific to your needs.

INTRODUCTION

The human body is designed for movement—and it moves best with practice. As we age, we sometimes stop using our bodies to their full capacity and can lose some of our mobility. These losses are reversible, in more cases than not, even if the loss was the result of an injury or other complicating medical condition.

I work with people every day to help them recover their abilities. Through my work, I have identified nine benchmarks for maintaining mobility:

1. Posture

2. Lying on your stomach

3. Getting off the floor

4. The squat

5. Overhead reach

6. The plank position

7. Single-limb stance

8. Sit-stand test

9. Endurance tests

All of these can be done at home without special equipment. My goal is to provide a framework to be done alone although in some instances, assistance from a second person may be helpful. I describe how to do each benchmark test and what to do if you have difficulty achieving it. These are described as simple exercises to help you improve to the point that you can achieve each benchmark.

Regardless of the source of their health issues, I have been privileged to help older adults regain physical capabilities they had lost and show them how to maintain and improve their mobility. This is true no matter how debilitated they were when I met them. The human body has remarkable healing and adaptive capabilities.

These regained abilities allowed them to live a more independent life—one that gave them hope and freedom to do more of what they choose to do. This is my love and passion—to give people the means to enjoy their lives more fully and with improved physical abilities.

As a physical therapist in a hospital setting for the past 10 years, I have had the opportunity to observe persons in a variety of conditions. Some enter with apparently no additional medical conditions to add to their primary diagnosis—the one that landed them in the rehabilitation hospital (be it a traumatic brain injury, spinal cord injury, multi-trauma from a motor vehicle accident, etc.). In other cases, older adults come with a laundry list of medical conditions.

These conditions can result in the necessity to consume an expensive cornucopia of medications, sometimes more than 20. The likelihood of medications interacting with each other is high. These interactions can lead to side effects, including the following: fatigue, drowsiness, constipation, cognitive dysfunction, sleep disturbances, anxiety, muscle weakness, balance impairments, and a myriad of others.

This condition in which persons are receiving long-term medical intervention, in an effort to manage their disease conditions, is indirectly "advanced life support." Without this medical supervision and intervention, they would surely continue to worsen. The medication side effects can be difficult to distinguish from the medical conditions themselves, in many cases.

You may already understand the above scenario if you were motivated to pick up this book. You have taken a particular interest in searching for answers to prevent this scenario from occurring or to improve your current condition. Although this book does not address general wellness for keeping the systems in your body operating maximally and optimally, it does address the components of movement and mobility that I feel are most crucial for the older adult.

SIMPLE SOLUTIONS FOR INCREASED MOBILITY

The tests and exercises I prescribe are in general simple things people can do at home with commonly available household items for tools. While some of these may appear to be common sense, they are in fact safe and effective ways to improve your physical capabilities and your mobility.

So many older people could avoid falling and avoid losing the ability to do common daily tasks with a little instruction and motivation. I wrote this book to reach more people, and to reach them before they need the services of a physical therapist to recover from injury or illness. I wrote it to help people regain and maintain their physical capabilities well into their old age, to offer them a better quality of life.

A deeper, more intensive study is required to understand how to optimize your overall wellness. There is a wealth of knowledge from experts in all areas, including nutrition, cognitive function and mental health, spiritual healing, and countless others. What I offer is designed to help you regain and maintain your physical capabilities, and these other aspects of health and wellness will also help you to maintain those capabilities. I touch on some of these aspects with some general health and wellness guidelines at the end of the book.

I hope this information is delivered in an easy-to-apply format. As I was deciding on how to present this information, I researched other resources on this topic, written for the older adult audience. The information and method of presentation were daunting, to say the least. Textbook after textbook came up, each with 300-plus pages, a thesis-worthy list of references, medical jargon, and an objective to cover all possible scenarios in their entirety and completeness.

I concluded that I personally would never get started with a program if I had to sift through that much material. I would be stuck in the perpetual vortex of wondering what to do and if it was working. I'd be changing my approach with every chapter I read until I never focused on a single area long enough to make a difference.

I decided on a short "manual" format in an effort to simplify the process and complete the objective: getting the older adult started, taking action, and moving forward *today*. You can review this material in its entirety in less than an hour. I know this because I frequently do this verbally with my older adult clients. A typical appointment lasts 60 minutes, and at the end of that 60 minutes, I generally send a person out with a small handful of activities to begin with, including postural reeducation, balance training, and a functional strengthening component. I developed simple tests to determine where to start with each person that could also be a way for them to maintain their abilities.

THE BENCHMARKS FOR MOBILITY

As you complete the benchmark tests, I provide action steps in two different phases. The *Practice Phase* refers to activities for you to do preferably on a daily basis, to effect change. Think of these as you would exercises to "improve" your condition, requiring attention and dedication.

Once you have achieved the specific benchmark test with what you consider ease and success, I describe the *Maintenance Phase*. This is a less vigorous and less frequent assessment approach to ensuring that the benchmark test remains easily achieved.

Practice the exercises weekly and once you can achieve the benchmark, assess monthly. I always encourage continued improvement through the progression of exercises.

This book provides the knowledge you need to maximize your mobility at any age. I believe a proactive approach to maintaining your physical abilities and independence is needed as you age. Without active use, your muscles will likely atrophy and your range of motion will become limited to the point that you may become unable to perform basic tasks. Illness or injury can contribute to physical decline if the recovery process does not include exercises to regain what has been lost.

HOW I CAME TO FINISH THIS MANUAL

Due to completely unforeseen circumstances, it has taken me four years to commit to finishing the manuscript for this book. Life has been an interesting adventure. I refer to the changes in my own life as "chapters." My wife says life is like ever-changing seasons.

Shortly after starting this project, specifically December 21, 2015, I began experiencing a slight euphoric dizziness. By December 29, this evolved into facial droop and three days in the hospital. The conclusion was something related to an autoimmune assault on my brainstem and its connecting nerves. With time and a large amount of anti-inflammatory steroids, my symptoms resolved. I then returned to my traditional habits of pushing myself harder. Every time I went back to my old ways, instead of achieving peak performance, sadly and unexpectedly I would crash and burn. I would be faced with an onslaught of new symptoms that eventually forced me into a six-week leave of absence from work and the inability to drive due to my dizziness and double vision.

During those six weeks, I took time to focus inward, to understand who I was and try to understand what was happening. It was a beautiful period of introspection. I learned two very important things: 1) I am not as resilient as I thought I was, and 2) no matter how "prepared" I try to be, life has a way of showing me how little control I actually have. It also made me a more empathic physical therapist.

Since then, I've dealt with residual deficits in my left eye and have a new perspective in life. I have continued my passion and work in helping people achieve more independence. My relationships with my children are richer, deeper, and more loving than ever. My love, respect, and appreciation for my spouse grows daily. I realize now that life *is* like the changing seasons: some harder than others, but with consistency, persistence, and courage, eventually the season will change. This idea reinforces my belief that being the most functional you can be and maximizing your mobility will ensure that you are best prepared to weather any storm life sends your way.

Completing this book has been a part of my reaffirmation that I want to spread my knowledge to more people than I can see in my clinic and continue my work in helping others regain and maintain their mobility. Do the best you can with what you have and recognize that you have the power to do this for yourself.

CHAPTER 1

The Posture Police

Physical therapists are known by many as the "posture police." Our family members, friends, and clients are all subject to our frequent observations and cuing to "stand tall," "squeeze your shoulder blades," "tuck your bottom in," and other forms of encouragement (or beratement, in some cases!).

As you age, the gradual decline in your balance is related to a number of factors—the benchmarks—covered in this manual. No factor is as important as posture. Your posture can fail for a number of reasons: decreased strength, pain, decreased range of motion, and lack of awareness.

Gravity is persistent. From the moment you get out of bed in the morning to the moment you lie back down, and until the day your ticket is punched, gravity is pushing you downward and in most instances, forward. With this perpetual forward shift of your center of mass, your tendency to lose your balance increases. Without the ability to correct this loss of balance, a fall and potential injury is inevitable.

One of the worst outcomes for an aging adult after a fall is a fractured hip. Disability and mortality increase substantially in many cases.

The first step to taking control of your independence is to develop the ability to have good posture. This doesn't mean you have to be in what would be considered "good posture" all the time. The only bad posture is a sustained posture, regardless of its approval. Sitting for prolonged periods is a sustained posture. That's why mobility experts recommend that workers get up from their desk and walk around a bit every hour. This is to change postures, joint positions, and increase motion, blood flow, and tissue health at joints.

BENCHMARK #1: POSTURE

Let's introduce the benchmark concept. A benchmark is a standard you test yourself against to determine if you meet the requirement. In the cases in this book, you either meet the requirement or you don't. If you meet the requirement comfortably and effectively, you can be "off the hook until next time." If you don't, you must incorporate tasks that help you to recover your ability, until the benchmark becomes easy to complete again. I recommend testing your benchmarks monthly.

Each benchmark requires a setup—the space and "tools" you need to complete it. These are simple things you will already have in your home, in most cases.

SETUP

For this benchmark, first locate a blank wall to stand against. A door would suffice. The most important thing is to make sure you have enough space to stand from head to toe, flat against the wall. There should be no pictures, coat hangers, window frames, etc.

Also, the flatter your foot position, the more optimal. Wear flat-soled shoes or go barefoot during the assessment. Avoid boots or shoes with tall heels, as this will drive your knees forward during the assessment. As a side note, use of tall heels will shorten your calf muscles and can lead to long-term changes that can affect alignment and posture, and result in pain all the way up to the low back.

PROCESS STEPS

1. Turn your back to the wall. With your feet as wide apart as your hips (legs straight up and down, not too wide), place your heels

against the wall. This is your first anchor in this activity. Your feet should grow roots in this position and not move from here.

Emphasis here on heels against the wall. The further they are away, the less effective this test is.

2. Make sure your buttocks come in contact with the wall.

    I've had some clients argue, "What if your buttocks are too large?" No matter the size of your backside, this is going to be the second anchor point. Once this occurs, make sure your knees are straight between the feet and the pelvis.

    Occasionally, people will bend their knees as they stand up more vertically with their trunk, which allows their pelvis to rotate due to restrictions at the hips. Not correct. Keep your knees straight.

3. The third step is to touch your shoulder blades to the wall. This is where people start having difficulty. As they attempt to stand more vertically against the wall, the tightness of the tissues on the front of their body begins to limit their mobility.

4. The final step is to touch the back of your head to the wall. If step three didn't cause a problem for you, this one may (it usually gets a large number of my clients). Do not make the mistake of looking up, extending the neck, and touching the top of the head to the wall. You must keep your eye level horizontal, your chin down, and pull the back of your head to the wall.

That's it! The benchmark for posture is that easy.

Now, let's talk about why and how we use this test for lifelong mobility.

Posture is essential to optimal control of your center of mass (your center of mass is your body weight balance point, generally positioned below and behind your belly button, though this varies with body type). Foremost, as people age and as your head is pulled forward due to gravity, you may increase your tendency to look downward. Looking downward may seem effective in ensuring that your every step is safe and steady, but it can cause your balance system within your inner ear to become less sensitive to gravity, or to interpret incoming information in a different way than intended. Over time, this can lead to further degradation in your "internal gyroscope," leading to declining balance and increased potential for falls.

In addition, as the tissue on the front of your neck shortens and weakens over time, and the tissue on the back of your neck lengthens and also weakens, the stabilizing effects of the miniature muscles between each vertebra in your neck lessen. This results in poor control of the individual bones, redirecting pressures to areas not designed for this task. Nerves become compressed, irritated, painful, and over time can cause further weakness.

Let's move down the spine. Prolonged forward flexion of the trunk, specifically the chest/ribcage and lower spine (lumbar spine), results in similar changes. Muscles and ligaments on the front of the body shorten, weaken, and pull forward. Muscles and ligaments on the back of the body lengthen and weaken, making them susceptible to injury. Pressures move to the front of the spinal column, and as bones weaken, this can cause injury, commonly referred to as compression fractures of the *vertebral bodies*—the areas designed to carry the load of your upper body and all you carry with it.

Shortening of the tissues on the front of the hips pulls on the low back. You may experience discomfort caused by this when trying to lie flat on your back in bed, or on your stomach. These muscles, specifically the "psoas," strongly attach into the lower lumbar vertebrae, and when stretched, pull hard on these vertebrae. With the back muscles in a weakened state, it can pull so hard as to cause movement forward, resulting in low back injuries and pain.

With tightness from above, the hamstring muscles on the back of the thighs are always working to stabilize. You may think this is good, strengthening these muscles. However, in reality they are overloaded continuously. Eventually they fatigue, reducing stability and opening up the door for injury.

Finally, moving down your body to the calf muscles, your foundation that meets the ground and secures your upright position. As described earlier, shortened calves caused by routinely wearing tall heels not only change the way the 26 bones in your feet move and the stress applied to the connections between them, but also affect the forces "up the chain" occurring at the knees, hips, and spine. It is not uncommon for therapists to find low back pain caused by the mechanics of the foot being "off," and correction alleviates the ailment.

HOW TO PRACTICE

If you find this benchmark difficult to maintain or are unable to get to the desired finished position, you need to work on it. You should practice regularly, frequently, and wholeheartedly. If you're a numbers person, practice at least three times daily for 5-10 minutes each time. Schedule your practice with your meals as an easy way to remember to do your activities. For example, you should perform your exercises/activities before or after each meal. That way, you have a cue in your environment that reminds you to complete your program in its entirety.

When you are able to achieve the desired finished position and it has become easy and comfortable to hold for sustained periods, you can move from the *Practice Phase* into the *Maintenance Phase*. Now you can back down from the intense practice and perform once a week, or even once a month.

When you begin performing once a month, you are truly using it as a *benchmark* because you are not getting any benefit from practicing it this infrequently. At this point, you are testing yourself to ensure that you are able to complete the task. If things become difficult again, or you find you are unable to get to the position described above, it's time to get back after it.

PRACTICE MADE INTERESTING: WHAT TO DO FOR IMPROVEMENT IN BENCHMARK #1

If you need to practice in order to achieve this benchmark (no such thing as shame here), here are a few postural corrective activities to make it interesting. These exercises not only will help to improve your mobility but will strengthen the appropriate muscles to correct your posture and protect your spine.

CORRECTING YOUR POSTURE

These practice exercises can be done as you stand against the wall in the same setup as for the benchmark:

» Place a tennis ball behind your head and press back into it. Try to hold it as long as possible. Set a timer, and always try to improve your time. If you can hold it for more than three minutes, you need to move to smaller objects (a piece of foam or a small paperback book) that allow your head to be closer to the wall.

» Have your partner place a fist or flat hand behind your head, or a flat hand behind your shoulder blades. Try to press back into it. This not only takes up space between the back of your head and the wall, but also cues you as to whether or not you're doing it correctly. You should feel the pressure of the hand as your head or shoulder blades compress it against the wall.

» If you have more restrictions and find that you can't get your shoulders to the wall, place a tall-back chair or walker in front of you. Use the handles of the walker or the back of the chair to lift your trunk up and extend your torso toward the wall. Early on, this may be necessary until you develop the range of motion and strength to get yourself there on your own. Repeat this regularly, and hold for 30-60 seconds, as tolerated. There is no magic number of repetitions or duration of holding. The main point is to practice frequently throughout a daily routine. The rule of thumb I give clients is this: "Treat it like mealtime. Once after breakfast, once after lunch, and once after dinner."

MOBILIZING YOUR SPINE

In addition to the postural corrective activities at the wall, you may also need to work on mobilizing your spine. Here are some safe and effective ways to gradually mobilize your spine:

» Start by rolling up a hand towel to make a compact cylinder shape. A general rule of thumb would be two to four inches in diameter, similar to the diameter of a hockey puck. You will use it in both the lengthwise and crossways directions. Place it on a flat surface, such as your bed, or on the floor for more support. Lie on top of the towel so that lengthwise, it runs the length of your spine. This specific technique allows your shoulders and chest to open into an optimal posture position. A specialty device referred to as a *foam roller* can also be used. However, foam rollers are a larger diameter (generally 6 inches) and may not be comfortable (as they are made of a firm foam and will not compress as easily). Stores also sell *1/2 foam rollers* (split lengthwise with one side flat and the other convex/rounded) that may be a happy medium. These look like a half moon from the end; not shorter, just smaller. I always look for things you have around the house first before sending you out to the store for equipment. You can easily progress from a hand towel to a bath towel and finally a beach towel folded lengthwise and tightly rolled.

» Additionally, you can use the towel roll crosswise at a variety of positions under your back to achieve spinal extension and mobilization at each location, as well as global extension across multiple locations of the overall spine. Start by placing the towel roll at mid-back, at the position just below your rib cage. Lie over the top of it to allow a stretch. Progressively move it up approximately two inches at a time to work on different locations up the spine. Many persons with posture issues find noticeable challenge with the towel roll higher, around the shoulder position.

Hold these positions for 30-60 seconds and repeat at mealtimes as described above.

IF THIS ISN'T COMFORTABLE . . .

If you are finding that the small hand towel causes pain or discomfort, you may choose to start with just lying flat on the firmest surface. You may need to provide a small towel roll or pillow for head support, initially.

Whenever positioned on your back, if you are feeling a strain in the hips and low back, this is a result of short hip flexor muscles and short, tight, sticky soft tissues on the front of the hip joint, lower abdomen, and front of thigh. **If you are experiencing more than a "mild discomfort" in this region and position, place your knees bent up, or a pillow/cushion underneath your lower legs.** This will reduce the stretch and strain on these tissues and make the position more comfortable and safer for your tissues and joints. The discomfort doesn't necessarily indicate injury and the need for medical intervention. Always look to progress to less support under the knees as you move toward optimal range of motion.

HOW TO KNOW YOU MAY HAVE OVERDONE IT

After any activity, my rule of thumb as to whether you've *overdone* includes the following:

1. New pain/discomfort lingers for an extended period of time

2. New pain/discomfort worsens after you stop the activity

3. New pain/discomfort limits your ability to safely carry out your mobility by making you feel imbalanced or weak and fatigued

When stretching, you should feel a mild discomfort but not pain. You could be overstretching if you begin to experience pain while stretching or immediately afterward. Stretching should result in feeling *good* after you finish.

Additionally, the activities performed with a towel roll can and should be progressed with overhead reaching, which is addressed later in the benchmark titled "Overhead Reach."

Many people are stunned as to their limitations initially when shown this benchmark activity and are inspired as they begin to notice changes in their posture. Usually, along with improvements in posture, they notice reduced strain and improved comfort through their low/mid/upper back and neck, increased ease of walking upright, and a renewed sense of confidence and vitality.

CASE IN POINT

Richard and his wife, Shirley, are aging adults, both in their 70s. Richard had a unique medical condition and he didn't have the energy to do the things he and Shirley enjoyed, including going for daily walks, traveling, shopping, and the like. Richard reported that he wanted to develop his energy, stamina, balance, and strength. Shirley wanted him to feel like he was able to do more throughout the day and engage more in life.

After we noticed his balance was mildly impaired and provided him with some basic exercises to work on, we tested his posture at the wall. He was able to get his heels, buttocks, and shoulders to the wall. However, he couldn't touch his head to the wall at all, not even when looking up. I recommended he keep his chin down, actively tuck his chin, and push his head back over his shoulders. As he practiced this, I encouraged Shirley to try the same. Shirley was able to effectively achieve the benchmark, however with difficulty and challenge. I encouraged Shirley and Richard to both practice this together as a mutually beneficial activity.

One week later, they returned for a follow-up assessment. Richard reported he was practicing daily. Not only had he improved his ability to get closer to the wall with the back of his head in a neutral position, he reported feeling like his posture was better, and his general discomfort had reduced with the exercise. As an added bonus, Shirley stated that the position was no longer difficult to hold.

Shirley felt their practicing was an activity that made her feel they were doing more together. Overall, Shirley reported that Richard was more active, they were walking daily, and he was feeling less fatigue from basic daily routines. With a comprehensive home exercise program of balance training, stamina development, and postural activities, Richard was more active, and he was happy with his reclaimed routine.

CHAPTER 2

The Dreaded "Face Down" Position

When was the last time you awoke to find you had been sleeping on your stomach? For many, in my experience, the answer has been "Not since I was a kid," or "Yes, in a previous life."

Lying on your stomach (I'm not suggesting sleeping on your stomach at this point) is extremely therapeutic and can work wonders for your range of motion and mobility.

Our society has moved from occupations with significant physical labor to jobs that require more sitting and less movement from the legs, hips, and trunk (as I sit and type this out). With prolonged sitting (day in, day out, year after year), what we don't realize is that we are slowly taking the shape of chairs.

As this happens, the tissues on the front of your body—such as hip flexors, pectorals/chest, abdominals, and muscles and ligaments that run along the front of your spine—shorten and become tighter and weaker. While this is happening, the tissues on the back of your shoulders, neck, torso, and low back become longer, looser, and weaker.

I routinely ask colleagues and physical therapy students the following questions: When is it appropriate for our spines to stop moving? What is the cutoff for when we should teach compensatory movements to older adults, versus teaching them normal movement that keeps those joints flexible and healthy?

I have grown to believe, and practice as my professional philosophy, that we should optimize the normal motion of the joints, stabilize that motion with muscles of proper length and strength, and allow the body to perform what it was designed to do: Our bodies are designed for *movement*.

BENCHMARK #2: THE DREADED "FACE DOWN" POSITION

Long story short, **lying on your stomach counteracts much of the negative effects of prolonged sitting.** Multiple, brief bouts of stomach time on any surface are effective.

SETUP

Lie flat on your back in bed or on the floor for a firmer surface.

PROCESS STEPS

1. Bend your knees up to allow you to roll onto your side, but don't start rolling yet.

2. Choose a direction for rolling onto your side, right or left. If rolling to the right, reach your left arm across your body toward the right and let your knees follow to the right, so you are lying on your side. (Do the reverse if rolling to the left. This process allows you to safely roll onto your side without twisting your spine.)

3. Once on your side, straighten your knees and hips, allowing you to roll to face down. Move the bottom arm parallel to your body to protect your shoulder, so you are not lying on your lower arm.

IF THIS ISN'T COMFORTABLE . . .

If you feel some strain in your low back in this position, that's alright. Don't be afraid of this position because of discomfort. However, if that discomfort becomes significant and unbearable, place a single pillow under your abdominal section. This will reduce the amount of extension at the hips and reduce the strain to the soft tissues and spine.

Similar to the posture benchmark, you either meet the benchmark of lying flat on your stomach comfortably, or you don't. If you don't, you need to practice.

If you have had a spinal surgery, consult a physical therapist or your physician before trying these practice exercises.

HOW TO PRACTICE FOR BENCHMARK #2

If you can't lie comfortably on your stomach and you need the pillow under your abdomen, you need to practice until this is easier and more comfortable.

THE PRACTICE PROGRESSION

» Lie flat on your stomach with a pillow underneath your abdominals. Once you can do this with no discomfort, try the next step with no pillow.

» Lie flat on your stomach without a pillow, face down or turned to the side, chest down on floor. When you can do this without discomfort, you are ready to start trying to arch your back in small increments.

» Begin to come up onto your elbows, keeping your hips in contact with the floor always.

» Begin to press up onto your hands, keeping your hips in contact with the floor always; if your hips begin to come off the floor, that is as high as you should go for that day. As a further note, not only will you gain movement of the tissues at the front of your body, but holding a position that keeps the hips on the floor without elbows straight will strengthen your shoulders, chest and arms. A double dose of benefit!

What does progress look like? Many people move from not being able to lie flat (requiring a pillow under the abdominals), to being able to press up into what yoga practitioners call the "cobra" or "sphinx" pose. This is a goal for everyone, because it not only demonstrates improved motion and flexibility throughout the spine and hips, but it improves the strength of the arms and shoulders as well.

TIME AND FREQUENCY

If you are dealing with tight, short tissues on the front of your body, spend 10-20 minutes on your stomach every day. When it becomes easy to assume and remain in the "face-down" position, then you can reduce the amount of time spent on your stomach. But I personally would not spend less than five minutes of dedicated time on your stomach daily.

CASE IN POINT

Charlie experienced a mild stroke that hospitalized him for two nights. He recovered rapidly and was quickly back to "normal." The discharging hospitalist recommended Charlie have a *physical therapy evaluation* to identify any subtle deficits, things the hospitalist couldn't evaluate. The doctor felt that a therapist could run Charlie through some standardized tests and tease out areas for improvement.

At first, Charlie said he felt "fully recovered," like nothing had happened. However, with some benchmark testing, he was found to have mild deficits in balance. Also, when we ran through the various functional positions (my benchmarks), he noticed he could not tolerate lying on his stomach without pain and discomfort in the low back. This was a long-standing deficit, not related to the acutely mild stroke he had experienced recently.

I recommended he practice a progression, using a pillow under the belly and then progressing to gentle press-ups. I didn't feel it was necessary to retest him on these areas, and recommended we have a follow-up phone call in three weeks to see how things were.

When three weeks came, Charlie reported that not only did his balance improve, but lying on his stomach was more comfortable. He said that because of this, he realized he hadn't been getting down on the floor to play with his two-year-old grandson. He had not realized what he was missing and he was incredibly happy with his newfound time with his grandson.

CHAPTER 3

The Rising Phoenix—Getting Off the Floor

A client once told me that her mother (who was well into her 80s) had the belief that getting down onto and up off the floor *every day* kept her independent. That statement was something I had always thought about, but this was the first time someone had reaffirmed it to me. It made me realize that people were interested in maintaining their mobility, willing to do something about it, and often just wanted a little direction.

The act of getting down onto and up off the floor is complex. People with mobility limitations struggle with it. It is considered a "necessary mobility skill" that is routinely taught to clients with debilitating neurological conditions. And when safely practiced and completed, it is one of the best, most comprehensive strengthening activities an individual can do to maintain their general mobility and "walk around" fitness. Also, being able to get off the ground is a pretty useful skill after a fall.

BENCHMARK #3: GETTING OFF THE FLOOR

If you cannot get up and down from the floor or it is very difficult for you to do, this is a critical benchmark you need to practice.

SETUP

Start by sitting on the edge of your couch or bed. Wear clothes you won't mind being on the floor in.

PROCESS STEPS

1. From this position, stand up, turn, and place both of your hands on the couch/bed so you are slightly bent over.

2. From here, step back with one foot and lower yourself into kneeling on one knee, with the upright leg being closest to the bed/couch. This position is what is called "half-kneeling."

3. Now, move to both knees down on the floor, or "tall-kneeling."

4. Move both hands to the floor, one at a time, until you're on hands and knees, or what we refer to as "quadruped."

5. From this "all fours" position, you can move to lying down on the floor.

6. Reverse these steps to get up from the floor. They are described again below, under "What to Do If You've Fallen."

This is helpful when carrying out a home exercise program or looking under the couch for your lost car keys.

The other thing to keep in mind is that throughout the above steps, you may find some components of the transition are more difficult than others. Spend more time practicing the more difficult areas. For example, if transitioning to/from half-kneeling is the hardest, spend more time working not only in this position, but transitioning to and from this position to strengthen your skills and abilities.

WHAT TO DO IF YOU'VE FALLEN

If you've fallen to the floor, your first and most important step is to take inventory of your status. Are you injured? If so, it may not be in your best interest to move. If you hit your head or have a broken hip, staying put is your best move. Use pain as your guide. As for hitting your head, if you feel dizzy, "knocked for a loop," etc., it would be best to have someone call for medical assistance if anyone is nearby.

If you are alone, you have no choice in the matter. You must get up and get to a phone to call for help. Often, lying in one position for too long can result in more damage than the fall itself. The body does not like inactivity, nor does it appreciate the pressure of lying on a hard surface for an extended period of time. This can lead to additional medical issues. So be prepared to get off the floor by performing the "Getting Off the Floor" activities. Practicing these as part of your benchmark activities will prepare you for an emergency and give you the confidence to know you are able to do them.

STEPS FOR GETTING UP OFF THE FLOOR

1. The first step is to roll over onto your stomach and then to your hands and knees, or to a position called "side-sitting," a position in which you are seated on your hip with your lower legs bent toward the opposite side, and your hands on the floor in front of your hips.

2. Either way, the next position is to move onto all fours (hands and knees).

3. On your hands and knees, you can crawl wherever you need to for safety. If you want to get off the floor, crawl to the nearest stable surface, approximately the height of a chair, couch, or coffee table.

4. Move your hands to the surface of whatever you intend to sit on next and assume the "tall-kneeling" position described in the benchmark process above.

5. Turn your body at a slight angle to the surface, with the side that you intend to lift yourself up with (your stronger, uninjured leg) closest to the edge of the piece of furniture.

6. Move into the position of half-kneeling. Bring your foot up so that it is planted firmly on the floor, while you remain in a kneeling position with the opposite knee farthest away from the surface you're moving to.

7. With your stronger leg poised to lift your body weight, lean yourself forward onto your hands and lift with your strong leg. The goal is to get your hips slightly above the level of the surface you are shooting for. You don't need to come to a full upright standing position.

8. Swing your hips onto the couch/bed/coffee table/etc. Voila! You have successfully gotten yourself off the floor.

OPEN WATER

What if you don't have a bed, chair, couch, or coffee table nearby? Say you fell in the mall, park, or grocery store. Then what?

Well, I'm not going to kid you. Getting off the floor in what I call "open water" (the space where nothing is near you that feels like safety, such as walls or furniture) is more difficult. This is where the practice is worth its weight. Practicing getting onto and off the floor on a regular basis will help improve your capacity to get off the ground in any situation, barring you haven't injured yourself.

HOW TO PRACTICE BENCHMARK #3

Practice in a situation where you are capable of getting down and back up. Remain near a chair, couch, or edge of your bed. Once you are on the floor, there are several activities to practice that will help improve your overall capacity. I describe exercises to be done on all fours, in the tall-kneeling, and in the half-kneeling positions.

ON ALL FOURS

From this position, the following exercises will improve your ability to get up and down. Note that the exercises are ordered from easiest to more difficult. If you can't tolerate an exercise in this progression or it is difficult to hold steady, then it is too advanced. At this point, you should scale back to a previous exercise. Before you begin, place a pillow under your knees if the surface is firm, your knees are painful, or you have had knee replacements.

» Practice shifting your weight side to side, through your arms. Shift to the limit of *your* stability, *your* comfort zone.

» You can also shift your weight through your legs, at your hips. This activity is called "wagging your tail."

» Alternate lifting a hand or knee off the floor, shifting your weight enough to get some air underneath it.

» Bend your trunk side to side, attempting to touch your shoulder to your hip. This will help strengthen the muscles on the sides of your torso, as well as help mobilize your spine.

» The "cow/cat" posture. Arch your back into the position of an agitated cat. Hold for five seconds, then allow your back to sag, like that of a cow or sway-backed horse.

» Alternate reaching with your arm out overhead in this position.

» Alternate kicking back with each leg, straightening it out as you lift it off the floor.

» Finally, the crème de la crème . . . Perform opposite arm and leg lifts at the same time. For example, while on all fours, lift the right arm out straight at the same time that you lift your left leg out straight. Try to hold this position for five seconds.

TALL-KNEELING

The position of tall-kneeling is when you are on both knees, with your hips extended and straight, and your torso upright. If you are able to assume and maintain this position without support, this will be the most challenging. However, if it is too difficult, have a chair/couch/bed or coffee table in front of you to place your hands on for support. The following activities can be done in tall-kneeling position:

» Shift your weight side to side, transitioning weight from one leg to the other.

» Kneeling squats: Move from an upright tall-kneeling position to sitting back on your heels. Return to the starting position. Avoid pain. Place a pillow or cushion between your heels and your buttocks to provide padding and support.

>> Alternate lifting one hand from the support surface.

>> Take both hands off the support surface but keep the surface in front of you for safety.

>> Perform one-arm exercises, such as side raises and front raises using a small weight (e.g., a soup can, brick, milk jug, etc.) or pulling on an elastic band from the front, performing back shoulder raises and rows with the elbow bent.

HALF-KNEELING

Move from kneeling on both knees to one knee down with the other foot planted on the floor. This would be similar to how athletes "take a knee" when their coaches are talking to them. Again, this is a versatile position as a lot of activities can be done here to improve stability, range of motion, and strength. Following is a list of some helpful half-kneeling activities:

>> Shift your weight forward onto the front foot, while keeping your torso vertical to achieve a deep hip flexor stretch. The pressure on the front foot should be felt through the heel or ball of your foot. Do not shift forward to where you heel comes up and the pressure is on your toes. Hold this position for a sustained time (30-plus seconds).

>> Maintain the position without hands on a support surface. This will help with balance, strength, and stability at the hips and torso.

>> Hold a gallon milk jug or lightly weighted object (under 10 pounds) in both hands, with arms extended out in front of you.

    a. If able, rotate side to side with the weight.

    b. Increase the distance you rotate each direction as you improve, but focus on comfort and stability, not how far you rotate.

» Perform one-arm exercises, as described under the "Tall-Kneeling" section.

A final suggestion is if you feel you do not have the capacity to get down or up from the floor safely, you should consider seeing a physical therapist to assist with evaluating this mobility deficit and teaching you effective techniques for conquering this task. There is nothing more valuable than the one-on-one training by a provider skilled in proper movement techniques.

CASE IN POINT

Mike came to see me after his first stroke. The stroke had affected the entire right side of his body, causing weakness and a reduced ability to plan and control movement (as a result of an injury to the area of the brain controlling his right arm and leg).

The initial goals of our work together were to help him recover his ability to get into and out of bed, stand up, and walk across the room. As he accomplished this, his wife, Lucy, mentioned she was afraid that if he fell down, he would not be able to get back up and she would not be strong enough to help him.

I was able to assess Mike's ability to get up off the floor by physically supporting him onto all fours on our mat table. I placed a chair in front of him and asked him to problem-solve getting up to the chair.

Through this assessment, it was clear he could not do this for reasons not exactly related to the stroke. He had limited range of motion due to tight hips and hamstrings, and a weak trunk and poor postural control. I attributed this to his lack of maintaining the capacity to not only get into but transition through the positions necessary to move from kneeling to standing, and then pivoting to the chair.

We first practiced moving from hands and knees to tall kneeling. We strengthened his stability in this position, then moved to assisted half-kneeling. Then, we continued to work on his ability to hold this position and increase his abilities while maintaining stability.

Soon, with training, he became more stable while transitioning between the necessary positions. Eventually he was able to move from hands and knees to upright tall-kneeling to half-kneeling, and finally lifting his hips and pivoting to a chair. For Mike and Lucy, this simple task development relieved their fears and helped Mike gain a sense of confidence he had not realized he was lacking.

CHAPTER 4

The Deep Squat

As children, when we're first learning to walk, we retrieve objects from the floor by squatting as deeply as possible. We are unable to bend forward to pick something up due to limited balance, trunk strength, and postural control. However, sooner or later, most everyone begins to bend forward to reach the floor, minimizing the amount of squatting they do. The required strength and range of motion declines as a person stops demanding it from their muscles and joints.

Whether you are able to complete a "deep squat" or not, the progression of activities below will help immensely with strengthening and balance, mechanics, and efficiency with getting out of a standard chair, something everyone needs to be able to do throughout their lifetime. If you are not able to achieve the deep squat as described, continue to the practice information and don't despair if you aren't able to achieve the full deep squat. The ability to do a partial squat still has value. Working towards it will improve your ability to stand up from a sitting position, which is critical to an independent life.

BENCHMARK #4: THE SQUAT

The goal of the functional squat is to get as low as possible without losing your balance and then return to standing without difficulty.

SETUP

Open floor, next to a piece of furniture or railing you can use for support if needed. The first time you complete this, place yourself in front of a low surface, such as a couch, for safety. Also, if balance is a concern with this activity, you can start by holding onto the back of a chair or couch to keep from falling backward. Wear loose clothing that will allow you full range of motion.

PROCESS STEPS

1. Place your feet slightly wider than your hips, with toes minimally turned outward. Keep your heels on the floor throughout the movement.

2. Start lowering your body into a squat, pushing your knees apart as you do this. Keep your center of gravity over your feet and do not let your knees come together as you squat. Your torso should remain as vertical as possible. The emphasis should be placed on controlling your center of gravity from falling back too far, while attempting to maintain verticality through the trunk and lower legs.

3. The lowest point of the squat should be with your hips below your knees (knee bend of more than 90 degrees), pain-free.

    Your knees should be aligned directly over or even slightly outside your feet.

A variety of cultures have maintained the ability to not only move into a deep squat, they also use it as an effective resting and functional posture. Here's how to restore your squat.

HOW TO PRACTICE: BUILDING UP TO THE SQUAT

Wear loose-fitting clothing while performing these exercises to allow you to comfortably move through the full motion without being limited by tight jeans or dress shirts.

» Start by using a kitchen chair, or similar setup, equipped with armrests. Start by standing in front of the chair as if you are about to sit down. Practice transitioning from standing to sitting in the chair, and then back to standing. Repeat for multiple repetitions until you feel fatigue (usually a burning sensation) in the muscles of the legs. My general rule of thumb is 10-15 repetitions continuously, without rest in between.

» As this becomes easy, progress to using a chair without armrests, placing the demand solely on your legs.

Additional suggestions: If you use an assistive device (i.e., cane or walker), determine the lowest surface you can stand up from and use a piece of tape to mark that same height on your cane or walker. That way, you will know if you are close when practicing on other surfaces. More importantly, you will know when a chair is *too low* for you.

SIT-STAND SEQUENCE

The sit-stand sequence is also an endurance benchmark and will be listed as benchmark #8 in a later chapter.

To move to standing, I always use the following sequence to achieve an optimal setup for safety, efficiency, and effectiveness:

Sit in a chair or bench, preferably with arms. An uncushioned surface is best.

FROM SITTING TO STANDING

1. Scoot forward until you are seated at the front of the chair/bench and you are unable to see the chair between your legs. You will still have a large portion of your pelvis positioned safely on the chair.

2. Move your feet back until your ankles are positioned **slightly** behind your knees. This doesn't have to be drastic, but subtle. An inch or so is enough to get the position correct.

3. Lean forward until your "nose is past your toes." Many people's difficulty with coming to a stand is that they do not get their center of mass (e.g., the central point at which the weight is equal in all directions) far enough forward.

    The majority of people I work with consistently lose their balance backward during a sit-to-stand maneuver. I encourage them to lean forward, looking down on their feet until they see that their nose is beyond their toes.

4. The cue I use is, "Take off like an airplane, not a rocket ship." The meaning of this is to come forward and upward at the same time, which moves your center of mass (your torso and hips, specifically) forward and over your base of support (wherever your feet are placed). When that occurs, only then are you optimally positioned to rise to standing.

    Taking off like a rocket ship suggests that the person attempts to stand without coming forward, moving straight upward from sitting. This places the center of mass behind the feet, making it impossible to safely and effectively transition to standing.

FROM STANDING TO SITTING

Moving from standing to sitting is simpler, as one would expect. Stand with the chair or bench you will sit on at your back.

1. As you begin to sit, actively push your hips back. Bring your shoulders forward at the same time so that you keep your chest held high. Visually fix your gaze on a point on the floor approximately five feet in front of you.

2. If you have safety concerns, instability, or difficulty, always reach back for armrests or the seat on your chair to ensure it is there, that it remains there (doesn't slide), and to help lower your mass.

   From this point, you understand the mechanics of transitioning from sit to stand and stand to sit. The best way to improve your capacity is to repeat, building strength and stamina through repetition. Frequently, I prescribe not only squats but repetitive sit-to-stand maneuvers from a surface for people to work on this capacity.

In addition to the above, remember to keep the following in mind when performing a squat:

» Try to always keep your heels on the floor, even in the lowest position.

» Keep your torso as upright as possible and focus your vision on a point on the floor five feet in front of you.

» As you squat down, keep your knees pushed outward to the sides (versus letting them collapse inward, indicating weakness at the hips).

ACHIEVING ADEQUATE RANGE OF MOTION

The lower you are able to effectively squat, the greater your functional capacity will be. You will be able to squat deeper to pick up objects safely and with improved ease.

The most important areas to work on are the ankles and hips. Typically, people have full range of motion at the knees, but may have weakness or pain.

IMPROVING HIP RANGE OF MOTION

To improve hip range of motion effectively and safely, perform the following stretches regularly.

» Lying on your back and keeping the opposite leg straight, bring one of your knees to your chest. You should feel a stretch in the buttocks region.

   a. You can hold for prolonged periods (30-60 seconds), or work to dynamically mobilize the tissue by pulling firmly, then releasing, and then repeating for 10 or more repetitions.

   b. Perform the same technique with the opposite leg.

» In the same position as above (on your back), draw your knee to your opposite shoulder to stretch the tissues on the outside of your hip. Perform in the same manner as the knee-to-chest exercise.

» Draw the knee to the outside of the hip to loosen the inside tissues, such as the groin and rotator muscles.

   a. If this becomes easy, bring the foot inward to achieve additional stretch to the rotators.

   b. Place the ankle of the raised leg on the opposite knee or shin, and let the leg fall out to the side. **Be careful with this motion if you have any history of hip surgery.**

» In "half-kneeling" (covered in further detail in chapter 3), place your back foot (attached to the knee placed on the floor) on a raised surface, such as a bolster, pillow, step, or block.

   a. Move your torso to upright to achieve a stretch on the front of your hip. Use a chair or dowel/PVC pipe for support.

   b. Hold this position for one to three minutes.

   c. Repeat with the opposite leg.

IMPROVING ANKLE RANGE OF MOTION

You will need access to a wall for these exercises. To improve ankle range of motion:

» Stand an arm's length away from the wall, facing it with both feet under the hips. Take one large step backward with one foot. This will assume a staggered or split stance position with your feet. The back foot is the targeted ankle.

   a. Place your hands on the wall for support.

   b. Bend your front knee while keeping your back knee and foot position straight. *Keep the back heel on the floor at all times.*

   c. Shift your weight forward onto the front leg to achieve a stretch in the back ankle and calf muscles.

» Also, if you have a small step (or you can do this against a wall), place your toes and ball of your foot against the step/wall, keeping your heel on the floor.

   a. Shift your weight forward and hold for 30-60 seconds to stretch muscles in your foot as well as calf. Hold onto a railing or stable surface as necessary. Repeat multiple times per day for optimal mobility of tissues.

IMPROVING HAMSTRINGS RANGE OF MOTION

To stretch your hamstrings:

» Lying on your back, keep one leg straight.

   a. Bring the opposite knee up, flexing the hip to 90 degrees.

   b. Lock your fingers behind the knee. Use your leg muscles to actively straighten the knee until you feel a deep stretch in the back of the thigh.

   c. Hold for two seconds, then release and repeat 10-15 times.

    d. An addition to this technique is to hold at the stretching point, and then pump your ankle up and down to loosen tissues throughout the back of your leg and foot.

Perform body-weight squats (no extra weights, just you) regularly to strengthen your leg and back muscles, while improving your squatting technique. You should practice additional squatting techniques described later under the chapter titled "Polishing."

CASE IN POINT

Meredith was a 68-year-old woman with a history of secondary progressive multiple sclerosis. She visited me after a recent series of falls. She had not been injured by the falls and was hoping to keep it that way.

Through our evaluation, we discovered that she had great difficulty standing up from any standard chair, including her manual wheelchair. When left to her own planning and execution, it was clear her center of gravity was not moving forward as she attempted to stand. She was holding her upper body and hips behind her base of support (feet on the floor). This was causing her to struggle to stand and resulted in her losing her balance backward. Also, when she attempted to squat, she would lose her balance backward.

We initiated the training with the succession of steps to effectively stand from a lower surface such as a chair. With a short period of practice, she understood her need to get her center of balance forward before "taking off like an airplane."

Once this was accomplished, we progressively trained her to control her squat deeper and more slowly by progressing to lower levels and then coming back up. With a short care plan of physical therapy and ongoing training and awareness, Meredith continued to develop her ability to not only stand from lower chairs in her home, but also to control her stability when retrieving objects from the floor in her environment. This made her feel safer and more independent in her life.

CHAPTER 5

Reaching the Top Shelf

Now that you have the tools to improve your posture and range of motion at your trunk and legs, it is important to address shoulders and arms to optimize functional capacity on a daily basis.

As we age, we tend to lose the ability to reach overhead. This is due to postural changes, reduced frequency of overhead reaching, and modifying our environment for ease of access. Because of this, shoulder capsules (the connective tissue that surrounds the joint and provides stability and lubrication), the chest muscles (i.e., pectorals, or pecs) become tightened, the stabilizing muscles of the rotator cuff (the muscles that provide the anchor for proper shoulder movement and active stability) become weakened, strength and joint range of motion become reduced, and the downward cascade perpetuates itself. After 10-20 years of changes in activity level, I often clearly detect decreased functional capacity for many people during my routine examinations. Most people don't realize how far they have declined until I point out these deficiencies. They are instantly surprised by their limitations.

With reduced strength and range of motion while reaching overhead, the potential for injury is increased, and many times people seek medical attention after developing shoulder pain or worse, a catastrophic injury while doing something like moving a paint bucket from the top shelf in the garage.

The good news is that this is preventable and routinely correctable. With a little regular practice and focused strengthening, you can maintain shoulder function throughout your lifespan. Let's discuss safe and proper techniques to achieve this.

BENCHMARK #5: OVERHEAD REACH

For optimal improvement, you must first be able to achieve the posture benchmark, #1.

Benchmark #5 uses the same setup. That being said, it is important to understand your limitations with this benchmark. You shouldn't wait until you achieve benchmark #1 before assessing and intervening with benchmark #5.

SETUP

Return to the wall as you were during the postural assessment (benchmark #1) and stand with your back to it.

PROCESS STEPS

1. First, achieve the position of the postural benchmark in standing, and then raise extended arms straight up above your head.

2. Attempt to touch your hands to the wall while keeping your elbows straight.

   A bonus would be to touch your elbows to the wall alongside your ears.

HOW TO PRACTICE: PROGRESSING TOWARD AND GAINING OVERHEAD FUNCTIONAL REACH

The setup for these practice exercises is variable—for some you will need to lie on the floor, for others you will need wall access. You will also need a five-foot length of closet rod dowel or one-inch diameter PVC pipe.

I like the PVC pipe best for the following reasons: 1) you can readily purchase a 10-foot length at your local hardware store for a fraction of the cost of the closet rod dowel, cut it in half and immediately have two lengths to share, and 2) as the closet rod dowel is used and ages, it becomes harder to clean and can cause slivers! The PVC pipe can be wiped down with a disinfecting cloth and you never have to worry about splintering.

Practice the following activities to increase your functional capacity for the overhead reach:

» Lie on your back on a flat surface.

a. While holding a dowel or PVC pipe in both hands with elbows straight, start by pressing it away from your body, toward the ceiling (perpendicular to your body's position, like a bench-pressing maneuver).

b. Next, reach overhead with extended elbows to allow gravity to assist with the stretch (in the direction parallel to your body).

c. Reach your maximal tolerated stretch (a mild discomfort of stretching in the soft tissues) and hold for 5-10 seconds. If you feel a "pinching" pain in the top of your shoulder, this is an indication the joint is being compressed (impinged), and you shouldn't stretch as hard. This will improve with the mobility of the shoulder joint with practice. Return to the starting position, indicated in point a).

d. Repeat multiple times (10-plus repetitions) to achieve sufficient stretching benefit and shoulder mobility.

» Stand less than an arm's length away from the wall, facing it.

a. Keep your body square to the wall; do not twist your torso sideways. Beginning with both arms directly in front of you (shoulders should be at 90 degrees to your body), walk the fingertips of both hands up the wall until you reach your maximum height. "Maximum height" is defined the same as in point c) in the above position, in which you experience a mild stretch without a "pinching" pain.

b. Hold at the top for 5-10 seconds. Then, slowly walk the fingertips back down.

c. Repeat multiple times (10-plus repetitions) with both arms.

» Place your back to the wall in the same position as the posture benchmark test. Hold a closet dowel or length of one-inch PVC pipe, approximately five feet in length.

a. Grip the pipe with both hands, slightly wider than shoulder width.

b. With elbows straight, bring the pipe upward in front of you as high as possible. Attempt to touch the pipe to the wall overhead.

c. Practice this activity by reaching as high as possible, holding for 5-10 seconds, then returning to the starting position.

d. Repeat multiple times (10-plus repetitions) to achieve sufficient stretch.

» Overhead press: Grasp the pipe at shoulder width with both hands.

a. Bend your elbows so the pipe rests on your upper chest, if you are able. If you cannot place the pipe in this location, a couple inches in front of your chest is sufficient.

b. Pull your chin back to clear the pipe as you attempt to press it overhead. Try to keep the pipe in a vertical plane. I cue clients to "try to touch the ceiling, making sure to get the elbows as straight as possible."

c. Hold at the top position for 5-10 seconds. Then return the pipe to its starting position.

d. Repeat multiple times (10-plus repetitions) to strengthen the muscles of the shoulder and upper arms functionally and effectively. Again, if you are feeling a "pinching" pain in the top of the shoulder, at the top of the movement, you should not press hard into this, as it is a sign you are impinging tissue, which is not optimal and can become irritating.

Using the equipment above to work on these techniques is sufficient and will ensure that potential for injury is minimal. However, once this technique is perfected, it would be appropriate to progress your capacity through increasing resistance by adding weight to the overhead-pressing maneuver.

Some recommendations for progressing the overhead press functionally are to use a gallon jug of water (50-100% filled for progressive resistance), a paint can, or a pipe with a cuff weight strapped to the center of it. This will allow you to measure your resistance and increase it accordingly. Other, more advanced and creative ways to increase resistance are to secure caps on the PVC pipe with pipe cement, and fill them with sand, cement, or another weighted material. These are relatively permanent, but if you have multiple PVC segments, you can create a series of progressive "weights" to complement a home gym.

A physical therapist or personal trainer would also provide additional direction and recommendation to maximize safety and success.

CASE IN POINT

Charlie was a 75-year-old man with a history of shoulder pain. He had made concessions for this by moving all of his items in the kitchen to lower levels so he did not have to reach overhead to get them.

He came to me after an acute medical condition, which was unrelated to the shoulder limitations. As I tested many of his systems, including balance, coordination, functional capacity, and movement patterns, I noticed that his posture and shoulder mobility was not optimal. I concluded that due to forward shoulder blades and tight and weak soft tissues, he had limited shoulder function and independence when reaching overhead.

Not only did we focus on increasing the normal movement of his shoulders, but as this improved, we progressed to strengthening. Over a short period of therapy and with a diligent dedication to the home exercise program I recommended for him (including rotator cuff strengthening, which will be discussed in a later chapter), Charlie began to feel less pain in his shoulders and was able to reach higher.

He discharged from my care with the newfound ability to retrieve moderately weighted objects from heights above his head. He reported that he felt able to grab appliances from higher shelves in his kitchen and had less difficulty pulling tools off shelves in his garage. His pain continued to improve and was no longer the limiting factor in his independence and ability to complete these new tasks.

CHAPTER 6

The Core

What would a book on wellness and fitness be without a chapter on the famous "core"? The core typically refers to the muscle groups of the abdominals and low back. However, I'd like to expand that definition to include the shoulders and hips.

Your four limbs (two arms and two legs) are attached to what is referred to as the "axial skeleton." This includes the spine, the pelvis, and the rib cage. The attachments include muscles and ligaments. The "shoulder girdle" (including the shoulder blade/scapula and upper arm/humerus) is attached to the rib cage by a group of muscles, primarily. The physiological purpose of this is to allow for maximal motion of the arm. However, because of this function of "maximal motion," this overall structure has the potential to be very unstable and susceptible to injury.

The leg is attached to the pelvis by a relatively deep socket joint at the hip. Ligaments, joint capsules and muscles help not only to hold this together, but promote proper movement inside the joint between the two bony surfaces. Though this joint is much more stable than the shoulder due to its direct bony attachment to the pelvis, with imbalances (weakness and tightness) come improper movements between the two bony surfaces. Over time, this leads to wear and tear in areas that are not designed to handle this "rubbing." The result is arthritic changes, tissue damage, weakness, and pain.

So, to reiterate, my definition of the "core" includes the muscles of the back (upper and lower), the muscles of the abdominals (four in particular, layered for maximal stability and control), the muscles of the shoulder girdle (the ones that hold the shoulder blade to the rib cage), the muscles of the shoulder proper (primarily the rotator cuff muscles that hold the upper arm to the shoulder blade), and the muscles at the front, side, and back of the hip joint (hip flexors, groin, and buttocks/gluteal muscle group).

We have a saying in my profession: "Proximal stability before distal mobility." Let me say that in plain English: in order to move the arms and legs safely and effectively, one must have a stable anchor point at the torso and pelvis. If the muscles of the trunk, including the shoulder girdle and hips, are weak and unstable, the movement will be sloppy, inefficient, and unsafe.

Not only is having a strong and stable anchor for movement important, also it preserves spinal stability and reduces the incidence of spinal injury and back pain. Imagine your spine being segments of a chain. As one segment moves to its limit, the next segment moves, and so on up the chain. Without proper stabilization from muscles, the excessive movement places strain on other tissues, such as ligaments and discs between the vertebrae. Over time, these tissues begin to break down and start "talking" to us. Pain and injury are the results, if we do not improve the support muscles.

In previous chapters, we discussed at length the importance of mobility of the spine. Previous sections provided suggestions for mobilizing the spine, such as lying on a towel roll and pressing up in prone position (chapter 3) and reaching overhead (chapter 5). Here, we want to discuss ways to stabilize once you have achieved the range of motion.

An analogy was once presented to me regarding the low back musculature: imagine your low back muscles and the surrounding, encapsulating tissue (i.e., fascia, which is like the marbling on a rump roast) are like a tent pitched in the wind. The poles act as muscle, providing structure, shape, and tension to the tent. Without maximal muscle presence and control, the tent flaps in the wind, eventually tearing and falling apart. Maintaining good strength and motor control of your spinal stabilizers, shoulder stabilizers, and hips will act as the tent poles, keeping the tent rigid and unwavering in the storm.

Before we get to the benchmark, we should discuss some very important muscle groups and how to engage them.

THE TRANSVERSE ABDOMINIS

The transverse abdominis, or TA for short, is the innermost layer of the abdominal muscles and belly wall. It runs horizontally when you're standing. It begins its attachment at both sides of your spine in the back of your abdomen, wraps around the sides, and attaches into the soft tissue of the "six pack" muscle, the rectus abdominis (that's the last of the jargon, I promise).

The TA acts as a corset. When activated, or cinched up tightly, it provides the wall of your abdomen with stability and control.

Not to get too far off track, but a wonderful expert in the field of cardiopulmonary physical therapy once described the abdominals as being the walls of a soda can. When the can is closed and under pressure, the walls are strong and unable to crush inward, giving stability to the overall structure.

When the TA is activated, it provides just that: a stable wall to serve as an anchoring point for purposeful movement. If the TA activates late, poorly, or not at all, the stability is compromised and injury is imminent. After a back injury, without proper retraining and rehabilitation, this muscle has been found to either turn on late in movement, or not at all.

So, how do you purposefully activate the TA?

There are a number of cues that can be used to activate the TA. My most common cue is to "draw your belly button toward your spine." Do not confuse this with "sucking in your gut" or taking a deep breath and then holding it. You should be able to gently tighten your TA and remain breathing.

The goal is to have the control of the muscle such that you are capable of engaging it whenever you want to or need to. Times when you need to include pretty much any movement, especially when lifting heavy loads or transitioning from compromising positions, including off the floor and out of bed.

BENCHMARK #6: THE PLANK POSITION

SETUP

Either lie on your stomach or get on your hands and knees. This can be done on any surface. If you are unable to get onto the floor, perform this on your bed (and return to chapter 3 to practice the necessary skill of getting onto and off the floor).

PROCESS STEPS

1. Have a timer ready or a second person timing your duration of this test.

2. Position yourself on outstretched arms, such as when assuming a push-up position. If you are unable to hold on outstretched arms (elbows straight), use a scaled-down starting point positioned on your elbows (elbows bent). It would be perfectly fine to put a soft layer of a towel or blanket under your elbows to reduce any painful pressure between the bony elbows and the floor/firm surface you are on.

3. The goal is to hold this position for 60 seconds or longer. During that time, make sure to hold your TA tightly by drawing it in and toward your spine. This will stabilize your low back during this and any other movements.

If you are capable of maintaining this position for 60 seconds or longer, you meet the benchmark. If you are unable to maintain this position for the required time, you have work to do.

HOW TO PRACTICE:
SUGGESTED ACTIVITIES FOR IMPROVING YOUR CORE

Though the title above indicates activities for improving your core, keep in mind that "proximal stability precedes distal mobility." The big picture is that we are interested in improving capacity at the shoulders and hips as well as with the abdomen.

TA ACTIVATION

» Lie on your back, with your knees bent up.

   a. Place your finger tips of each hand on the sides of your abdomen. Imagine a clock, with your belly button at 12 and your spine at 6. Your fingers should fall in somewhere around 2-3 and 9-10.

   b. Without taking a deep breath, pull/draw your belly button toward the spine, as if you are trying to squeeze into a tight pair of Levi's. You should feel the muscle activate under your fingertips. It may be subtle, or it may be strong.

   c. Hold this activation for 5-10 seconds, then slowly relax.

» You can add in posterior pelvic tilts while performing the above exercise.

   a. Lying on your back, with your knees bent up, you will feel a "void" underneath your low back, due to the natural curve of your lumbar spine.

   b. While engaging the TA, flatten your low back and press it into the floor. This will engage the rest of your abdominal muscles and teach you stability with your spine in a neutral position.

When turning the TA on and off, I use the following analogy: recall the stereo systems with the dial that turns the volume up and down? Imagine that as you engage your TA, you are turning the volume up from 0% to 70% of maximum volume. As you hold, you maintain it at 70%. Then, and this is crucial, as you release the abdomen, turn down the dial very slowly from 70% to 0%.

It is not uncommon to feel muscle "tiredness" on the sides of your torso, abdomen, and even deep in the low back as this muscle fatigues, given the nature of the muscle's position and attachments.

Complete 2-3 sets of 10-20 repetitions until you get good control over this.

BRIDGING

» Lie on your back with your knees bent up again, similar to the previous position. Feet should be flat on the floor.

    a. Place your hands on your abdomen, or for increased ease of movement, at your side.

    b. Press down through your heels and lift your buttocks off the floor.

    c. Only lift as high as you can without causing undue strain to your low back or neck. There is no need to raise up all the way if you cannot. Muscles of the hips, buttocks, and along the spine will be engaged and working no matter how high your hips are off the ground.

    d. Again, hold for 5-10 seconds per repetition, then return to the starting position.

    e. Complete 10-20 repetitions per set, and 2-3 sets per session.

PLANKING

» In many of these scenarios, the test and the task are one and the same. Practicing a plank position regularly is the best way to improve the stability of your torso, abdomen, and pelvis.

    a. Refer to the benchmark above for instructions on how to complete this task. Hold for up to 30 seconds. Remember, there is no magic number to hold. The longer you are able to hold in the correct position, the stronger and more stable you are becoming.

b. If holding with knees off the floor is too difficult, prop on your knees to reduce strain and improve stability, tolerance, and the ability to build stamina. Additionally, if holding the arms straight is too challenging, it is alright to start on your elbows. Remember the goal of holding with your elbows straight, as something you can improve toward.

SIDE PLANKING

» Assume a plank position on your elbows.

a. From this position, lift one arm and leg up and rotate yourself into a position where you are only propped by one arm and your legs are stacked atop one another.

b. Hold this position for up to 30 seconds.

c. Repeat on the opposite side.

THE TURKISH GET-UP

» The most important thing you can do is package up your strength and abilities into a functional activity. The Turkish-Get-Up is just that.

a. Lie down on the floor.

b. Holding one arm overhead, get up off the floor, moving from lying to side-sitting, to kneeling, to standing.

c. Then repeat the sequence in reverse.

d. Make sure to alternate which arm you are holding overhead.

Add resistance by holding an object in the outstretched arm (e.g., a can of soup, your PVC pipe, etc.).

A final note on the Turkish Get-Up is that this is a relatively advanced activity. Make sure you feel confident and comfortable when trying this. Having good balance and coordination is necessary, and it is alright to not practice this until you feel ready.

Richard was a 68-year-old man who came to see me after dealing with a long history of back pain. This resulted in a general decrease in activity level. Over time, Richard noticed that his balance felt worse. After discussing with his primary care physician, Richard received a prescription for physical therapy.

Over several visits, we determined a series of activities to promote balance retraining. I also noticed that when he attempted to hold a plank position, he was clearly unable to maintain the desired position for any longer than 25 seconds.

Additionally, he complained of back pain that increased with this exercise. When his transverse abdominis was assessed, he clearly could not turn it on sufficiently and hold it with any control.

With a progression of transverse abdominis exercises and a progressive planking program, starting with his knees on the floor and elbows straight, Richard was able to find core stabilization exercises that did not provoke his back pain.

As his abdominals and low back became stronger, he was able to maintain a planking position for much longer. With his back pain improved, Richard was willing and able to be more active in the community.

He returned to a community-based exercise program and was more than satisfied to know he had taken control of his future abilities with just a little attention to neglected and weakened areas of his body, especially his core.

CHAPTER 7

Balance

Balance is the interaction of three systems that results in your ability to maintain a body position, particularly sitting and standing. Those three systems are as follows:

» Your *vestibular system,* or inner ear, that tells your brain where your head is in space and if it's moving

» Your *proprioception,* or joint position sense, that makes it possible for you to touch your nose with your eyes closed, stand with your eyes closed, and walk to the bathroom in the dark

» Your *vision,* which provides visual input of your surroundings to show you where vertical lies

Balance can be trained in people with and without contributing medical conditions. However, the degree to which balance can be improved upon is related to certain medical conditions. Neuropathy, for example, results in not only weakness but lack of sensation in the lower legs and feet. The diminished sensation is not likely to change with balance training, though some new research is proving otherwise. That said, it is not uncommon for balance to improve with practice, regardless of the condition.

Though the three systems listed above contribute directly to balance, there are a number of additional factors that indirectly contribute. Those include strength, motor control (the ability to control precise movement), and range of motion (specifically at the ankles, knees, hips, and torso). Range of motion for these four areas were covered in previous chapters of this book.

Make sure you have addressed the benchmarks in the previous chapters so your balance is as refined as possible.

There are two types of recommended balance activities: *static* and *dynamic* balance exercises.

STATIC BALANCE ACTIVITIES

Static balance exercises challenge your ability to control your body while remaining still, with varying changes to your base of support and with input from your visual system. Below is a progression from easy to more difficult static balance activities.

» *Normal* base of support: comfortable standing with feet at hip width apart.

» *Romberg* base of support: bring your feet together so the toes and heels come in contact.

» *Modified tandem* base of support: one foot staggered forward and to the side of the other, no matter how far apart.

» *Tandem* base of support: standing heel to toe.

» *Single-limb stance:* standing on one leg while holding the opposite foot off the floor. At this point, it doesn't matter where the raised foot is held. The objective is to stand on one leg for a period of time, regardless of the position of the raised foot.

» All of the above while standing on foam: all of the above positions can be progressed by standing on foam, a cushion, or a pillow to increase the level of difficulty.

» Standing with your eyes closed: all of the above positions can be progressed by assuming the position, then closing your eyes. **(Note: this is extremely difficult to do in *tandem* base of support or *single-limb standing*. It would be wise to have someone standing close by for supervision while completing this.)**

SETUP FOR STATIC BALANCE ACTIVITIES

Find a corner in your home with accessible walls to practice these tasks. That way, if you happen to lose your balance, you can catch yourself by placing your hands out against the walls.

» Back into the corner until you are touching the walls on both sides. Take one medium step forward, so you are no longer supported by the walls but they are close enough to touch if needed. You may also place a chair with a high back in front of you if you find you are losing your balance forward.

   a. Choosing from the static balance activities list above, have someone time you, use a kitchen timer, or count in your head to measure your ability. For example, you may be able to stand indefinitely with a Romberg base but can only stand 15 seconds in tandem and three seconds in single-limb standing.

   b. Practice at the levels where you are deficient (in this case, more time should be spent at tandem, progressing to single-limb standing as your balance improves).

   c. Track your progress with a diary, described later.

BENCHMARK #7: SINGLE-LIMB STANCE

SETUP

Use the single-limb stance (see description above) while standing in a corner.

PROCESS STEPS

See the *single-limb stance* description above. Use your time as your benchmark, with a goal of standing one minute on one leg without losing your balance.

Most older adults can only spend a limited amount of time in this position. A good benchmark would be one minute and would ensure that you are maintaining high-level balance skills.

DYNAMIC BALANCE ACTIVITIES

Dynamic balance activities help you train to maintain your balance while moving a part of your body. Your ability to control your balance by reaching for an object at any height, turning your head to look for a car while crossing the street, stepping over and around objects in your path such as curbs, and changing directions abruptly to avoid running into the wall, as well as an infinite number of other scenarios, is crucial to your independent mobility.

A test that we complete to assess a person's dynamic balance includes the following tasks in sequence:

» Normal walking

» Walking while changing speeds

» Walking with horizontal and vertical head turns

» Start and stop walking by external influence (examiner cues subject)

» Stepping over and around shoe boxes and cones

» Walking heel to toe

» Walking with eyes closed

» Walking backward

» Walking on toes

» Walking on heels

» Stepping sideways

» Braiding (cross-over stepping front to back)

» Tapping foot on varying curb heights

» Negotiating stairs

Though each of the above activities contributes a specific element to dynamic balance, all address a variety of conditions that hone your mobility skills.

SETUP FOR DYNAMIC BALANCE ACTIVITIES

Identify an unobstructed length of hallway or sidewalk to practice these skills.

See how far you can walk and how well you complete it. Is it easy, or does it feel incredibly difficult? If it is difficult, it is an area that requires additional attention and time spent refining the skill.

ADDITIONAL THOUGHTS

Both static and dynamic balance activities can be practiced indoors as well as outdoors on what I refer to as "compliant, variable terrain" such as grass, gravel, inclines, declines, side-hills, and other commonly accessed areas. Whatever your goal is, it is important to practice in these environments to improve your balance and mobility under such conditions.

CASE IN POINT

Patricia was a 78-year-old widow, living alone. I met her when she began noticing a decline in her abilities as her Parkinson's disease progressed. Through appropriate testing, we found her balance to be moderately impaired due to the tremor and rigidity, which are common symptoms of Parkinson's disease.

I provided her with a variety of balance exercises including static holds and repetitive, dynamic stepping and walking activities.

After a few weeks of formal therapy, she reported that not only was her balance better, but she was doing more at home. Specifically, she noticed the change when she was vacuuming her living room and was able to get down on the floor and clean underneath her couch. Her daughter, who had been providing support over the years, said Patricia had not been this independent in quite some time, and said she was having to do less for her now. Both were grateful for the newfound independence Patricia was experiencing.

Sadly, years later, Patricia fell back under inpatient services as her Parkinson's disease progressed and she had a fall, fracturing her hip. Her recovery was challenging, and she did not recover her ability to live independently.

CHAPTER 8

Endurance and Cardiovascular Exercise

When we talk about lifelong function and mobility, we don't only look at the ability to move your body from one position to another in a single attempt. As important as that is, it is equally important to be able to repeat it whenever you desire. This is what is referred to as *endurance*.

There are two types of endurance. Both are slightly different in characteristic and capacity. However, they overlap somewhat in functional expression.

TWO TYPES OF ENDURANCE

The ability to repeat a movement, whether it be at low or high intensity is considered **local muscular endurance**. Examples of this are cleaning your cupboards, stacking paint cans, vacuuming, carrying lumber, etc. The ability to sustain an aerobic activity over a period of time is considered **cardiovascular endurance**. Examples of this are walking, running, cycling, or mowing the lawn continuously. Both types of endurance are equally important when it comes to maintaining mobility and functional independence.

BENCHMARK #8: 60-SECOND SIT-STAND TEST

This test was mentioned as a practice exercise for achieving the deep squat, in chapter 4. Here is a timed version that is an effective muscular endurance test.

SETUP

Start in a seated position.

PROCESS STEPS

1. When the timer starts, transition to full standing, then return to the starting position.

    i.   Repeat as many times as possible in 60 seconds.

    ii. Progress the level of difficulty by not using your hands to push from the armrests.

2. If you can do 20 or more repetitions, you are in good shape at any age.

MEASURES OF ENDURANCE

LOCAL MUSCULAR ENDURANCE

Some common recommended benchmarks for local muscular endurance include the following:

»   60-second sit-stand test as described in Benchmark #8 (above).

There are several variations on the sit-stand test that can be used for practice.

» 30-second sit-stand test: similar to the previous measure, only 30 seconds in duration.

» Five-time sit-stand test: similar to previous measures, only measuring how long it takes to transition from sit to stand and back, five times.

Beyond sit-stand tests, other endurance tests involve lifting activities such as the floor-to-overhead test:

» Floor to overhead: use a gallon milk jug filled with a predetermined volume. Start holding the milk jug at your navel.

   a. When the timer starts, squat down and touch the floor.

   b. Next, stand fully erect and reach overhead with the gallon jug.

   c. Repeat the full movement 10 times.

   d. Time how long it takes to complete the activity. You can use a medicine ball, paint can, or no resistance to substitute for the milk jug.

CARDIOVASCULAR ENDURANCE

Some common recommended benchmarks for cardiovascular endurance include the six-minute walk test, the 12-minute walk test, and the timed distance test. A minimum benchmark would be the six-minute walk test. You can choose one of the others as your benchmark if you want a more challenging test.

BENCHMARK #9: ENDURANCE TEST

SETUP

Six-minute walk test: identify a length of hallway or sidewalk of 60-100 feet. Place a marker (e.g., pop can, cone, etc.) to plot your course. If you have access to a walking measuring roller, I recommend using one for accuracy.

PROCESS STEPS

1. Start your timer and perform laps around the markers until the six minutes are up.

2. Count your laps, read your measuring roller, or rely on whatever you use to track your distance.

   i. Progress by increasing the number of laps you complete.

3. A benchmark walking speed of 2.7 miles/hour for a distance of 1435 feet is considered normal and average. To translate: this is approximately 1/4 mile and should take you 6 minutes to achieve.

More challenging endurance tests follow:

» *Twelve-minute walk test:* same as previous measure, only for 12 minutes as this more effectively measures cardiovascular endurance.

» *Timed over distances:* identify a distance, either indoors or outdoors. One client used the distance from his home to the cattle guard down the road. He measured how long it took him to walk to the cattle guard and back, and always worked to improve his time. Other examples include number of houses or blocks.

HOW TO PRACTICE

In many instances, the tests are how you practice. In other words, improving your 60-second sit-stand test can be done by practicing sit-stands under a timed condition. If you want to improve on a six-minute walk test, walk as briskly as you can for six minutes and keep track of the number of laps you complete so you can improve each time you do it.

EXERCISE GUIDELINES

That being said, I have also included some recommended guidelines for cardiovascular exercise.

A person should participate in 20-60 minutes of cardiovascular activity five out of seven days per week. That seems highly variable, ranging from a minimum of 100 minutes to a maximum of 420 minutes. I always recommend that you work up to 30 minutes of cardiovascular exercise most days of the week. This could be in the form of brisk walking, hiking, jogging, cycling, or whatever your heart desires.

Evidence suggests that 30 minutes can be *cumulative*. This means your benefits are about the same if you participate in three bouts of 10 minutes' worth of activity or 30 minutes continuously.

CASE IN POINT

Ron was an 80-year-old retired principal of a large rural region of grade schools. He had a long-standing history of a nerve condition that resulted in weakness and arthritic joint deformity at the knees.

We met after he underwent a reverse total shoulder arthroplasty, in which his shoulder joint was replaced. His walking was limited by weakness, balance deficits, and pain in the knees. Using exercises from this chapter, he improved his basic mobility skills over time and he was discharged home.

Over a series of outpatient sessions, he continued to improve. We helped the knee condition by providing supportive bracing. At the time of discharge, it was recommended that he walk with his four-wheeled walker to the property fence at the end of the dirt driveway and back on a daily basis. It was also recommended that he time this distance and monitor whether he was improving on his speed and tolerance.

Over time, Ron reported that not only did he see a decrease in the amount of time it took to get to the property fence and back, he felt much more confident, safe, and capable. He had independently increased his frequency to multiple times per day, and felt his stamina and strength improving.

The last time I saw Ron was at a charity event, and he had also undergone a knee replacement to improve the alignment of his knee. He stated that the pain was "night and day" better, and his balance and independence was better than it had been in years. He was socializing and walking around the event without any support from a walker or his wife, and he felt safe. Also, he hadn't had any falls.

CHAPTER 9

Polishing

Once you have made it to this point in the manual, I expect you have begun implementing the activities from the chapters before and hopefully are noticing changes.

There are a number of ways to go about increasing strength and function, from many different philosophies. There are also a few wrong approaches that can leave you at risk for injury. Each approach has some very important keystones that make it work.

THE MOST IMPORTANT WAY TO PRACTICE

The critical message I want to communicate is the importance of continued movement. If you keep moving, you will maintain your range of motion, functional strength, and motor control. You will also experience less pain. If you add weight in the form of body weight, free weights, and gravity, you implement resistance training. Resistance training is essential to increasing muscle strength and functional capacity beyond your current state. Resistance training has also been shown to be an effective activity for improving bone density and tissue health.

This chapter is focused on techniques and ideas that progress and improve some of the functional skills discussed above, safely and effectively. The objective is not to identify your maximal strength production, but to challenge your body to function in a variety of different demanding postures and positions.

WEIGHTED SQUAT

» Once you have mastered the deep squat, the next progression is to add resistance to the movement. You do not need to load a barbell on the back of your shoulders and squat like a power lifter. But I am suggesting that you add overload to your system in order for it to respond, grow, and build itself up.

    a. Pick up a milk jug and hug it close or put on a backpack with 5-10 pounds added to it. Note that a backpack on your back will move your center of gravity/mass backward, putting you at increased risk of losing your balance backward. Sometimes, I recommend putting the backpack on the front of your body, keeping it close to your chest, similar to holding the milk jug.

OVERHEAD SQUAT

» As we discuss functional movements, specifically the squat and the overhead press separately, integrating them together applies an additional challenge to the nervous and muscular system. The overhead squat has a variety of benefits, including improving demand on postural, upper extremity, and lower extremity muscles during the squatting activity.

    a. Grip your PVC pipe with a wide grip. The cue I use for the wide grip is to assume as wide as required to naturally hold the pipe at your hip crease (the hip crease is where your legs meet your pelvis on the front of your body).

b. Lift the pipe to the overhead position, with the shoulders flexed as far as possible. An ideal position is to have the arms behind the ears.

c. Keeping the torso as upright as possible and the knees pressed apart, squat to the deepest position safely possible. The pipe should remain in a vertical plane and be positioned directly above the back of your head.

d. If the pipe drifts forward, this is caused by a lack of range of motion or stability in the shoulder joints. To improve stability of the pipe overhead, focus on pulling the pipe apart through its length.

e. A strategy for improving shoulder, arm, and pipe position at this moment is to widen your grip on the pipe.

f. Return to the upright position, pressing through your heels as much as possible.

» An alternate position for the overhead squat would be to place your hands behind your ears. For this technique, you are not using the PVC pipe.

FRONT SQUAT

» The front squat requires gripping the PVC pipe at a slightly wider grip than shoulder width. The pipe should be placed on the front of the shoulders, resting on the upper chest with the elbows pressed as high in front of you as possible.

a. From this point, squat down by pushing your hips back and lowering your buttocks to the deepest position comfortably tolerated. If you desire, place a chair behind you and squat down until you touch the seat.

b. Press up from this position through your feet and heels. Keep your torso upright to maintain the PVC pipe in its appropriate position. Keep the PVC pipe resting on the shoulders as able.

c. If you are unable to keep the PVC pipe resting on the front of the shoulders, another technique for proper form is to cross your arms across your chest without the PVC pipe.

DEADLIFT MANEUVER

» Whenever someone retrieves an object off the floor, whether it be a sack of groceries or an Olympic barbell, the technique should be the same. You are safest and most functional when you use your legs and not your back in this maneuver.

a. Stand with your feet slightly wider than your hips, toes pointed straight ahead or minimally outward (one o'clock on the right, 11 o'clock on the left).

b. Hold your PVC pipe at waist level so your hands are slightly wider than your hips. Your chest should be held high.

c. Tighten your abdominals and keep your back in a flat, neutral position.

d. Begin the exercise by pushing your hips backward and bringing your chest forward. Do not bend downward at the trunk by rounding your spine. The PVC pipe should remain in a vertical plane.

e. Lower the pipe by bending at the knees. Your trunk will bend forward slightly.

f. As the pipe reaches the knees, push your knees backward to clear the pipe. Let the pipe move in a vertical plane close to your thighs and shins, directly above your feet.

g. After the pipe passes below the knees, allow the knees to come forward. The heels should remain on the floor throughout the movement.

h. The lowest position is variable, but I encourage you to attempt to place the PVC pipe mid-shin. Your torso should remain upright as much as possible and should flex forward no more than approximately 45 degrees. Your spine should be held in neutral. Tighten your abdomen and low back to maintain this. Visual focus should be on a point on the floor approximately five feet in front of you.

i. As you push to return to upright, imagine pressing the earth away from you through your heels. Visualize drawing the PVC pipe vertically up your shins until it reaches your knees. Simultaneously, push your knees back to clear the PVC pipe. Emphasize driving your hips forward as you come to upright.

j. Finish with your chest held high and the PVC pipe at the level of your hips. It is unnecessary to hyperextend, or arch, your back (leaning backward when standing, accentuating the curve of your low back) at the top position.

LUNGE

» The lunge position reduces your base of support and increases the demand placed on your legs. You will need an open floor space and a towel or blanket to place under your back knee, in case it touches the floor.

a. With a comfortable stance, place your hands on your hips.

b. Step forward with your right foot as far as you comfortably can, so that you are standing in what I call a "split/staggered stance." To increase stability, widen your stance side to side, not front to back.

c. From here, lower your hips, keeping your torso upright throughout the exercise. The front knee should bend to near 90 degrees and the back knee should have minimal bend. To protect it from injury, do not touch the back knee to the floor, but lower it as close to the floor as possible. Place a folded towel or blanket under it to soften any contact.

d. Attempt to keep your hands at your hips throughout the exercise. Press through the front leg to return to upright. Step back to the starting position of feet side by side, then repeat with the left leg.

One thing to keep in mind is that in the lower position, the front knee should not be in front of the toes, but directly over the ankle joint. Keep the heel on the floor as much as possible. The pressure should be felt through the ball and heel of your front foot. If you are finding this is difficult, move your front foot forward more.

CLEAN AND JERK PRESS

No matter what the object is, there is no more effective or efficient technique for moving it from the floor to overhead than the clean and jerk press. This technique incorporates the *power clean* (a way to lift an object from the floor, used by weight lifters) with the *jerk press,* both commonly observed in Olympic lifting. Fear not, you will not be working toward an Olympic gold medal, but toward a more functional capacity to move normal household objects overhead.

The utility of this capacity is evidenced in my personal life when in my garage: stacking tires, moving boxes and paint cans to shelves, picking up my daughters and lifting them into the air, and countless other routine tasks. With a little practice, this exercise will increase your ability to routinely manage daily chores.

» Begin by holding the PVC pipe at the level of your hip crease, as previously described.

» Begin the exercise as you would with the deadlift maneuver, lowering yourself to the bottom of the lift with both knees bent.

   a. From the lowest point, press up with your legs as you would in the deadlift maneuver. When the PVC pipe reaches mid-thigh, this is where the technique changes.

   b. The objective is to use leg power to thrust the pipe upward. The greatest power generation comes from your legs and hips, so you want to maximize their output. This drives the PVC pipe upward.

   c. Immediately after the drive upward, the next step is to drop your hips (ideally, you must bend your knees here to do this but it's alright if you can't, initially) sufficiently to allow your arms to rotate under the pipe, catching it on your upper chest, similar to the starting position of the overhead press.

   d. Straighten your knees to a fully upright position, with the pipe still held at your upper chest.

   e. Next, press the PVC pipe overhead like described in the "Overhead Press" section of the chapter "Reaching the Top Shelf." Finish with your arms extended overhead.

   f. For heavier objects, squat approximately 2-3 inches, then thrust from the hips to move the object overhead.

This exercise can be progressed and modified to use a number of objects. Commonly used items are a dowel/PVC pipe, medicine ball, one-gallon jug of water, paint can, or even a basketball.

At this point in the chapter, it is important to say that these exercises have been derived and incorporated from an industry of human performance enhancement, such as is found in the fitness industry and the area of competitive sports. All of these exercises are keystone across the board, as they are foundational strengthening and power-producing maneuvers. They can be safely and effectively incorporated into application for the older adult.

If you desire to progress these beyond the intent of this manual, which is the functional application for improved general capacity and maximum mobility, I encourage you to identify a professional resource in your community. Strength and conditioning experts as well as physical therapists with specific training in the area of athletic performance enhancement are perfectly capable of instructing you to apply resistance loads to these exercises safely and effectively. More philosophy is discussed in a later chapter.

CHAPTER 10

General Health and Wellness Guidelines

The previous chapters addressed movements necessary to achieve sufficient motion, mobility, and functional capacity to carry out normal, daily activities. Once you are able to complete these or become proficient at going through the movements, it is perfectly satisfactory to stop there and use the benchmarks provided at each chapter to determine maintenance of function.

However, many older adults desire to continue to grow, progress, and improve their overall capacity beyond the basics. Keep in mind that being strong, having the ability to generate power, and having optimal range of motion contributes to many positive direct variables of function. In other words . . . these abilities can allow you to do many satisfying and fun activities.

Strength improves function. The stronger a person is, the more capable they are to move their body, manage and carry loads, and manipulate objects.

BENEFITS OF GREATER STRENGTH

In most instances, improving strength of the muscles around a joint results in decreased pain at that joint. Frequently, pain at a joint is thought to be caused by the degraded surfaces of bone within the joint, which is referred to as osteoarthritis. However, when people apply a progressive strengthening program, the pain improves and frequently resolves.

This is thought to be related to a number of factors: strength in the muscles surrounding a joint improve stability of that joint. This prevents excessive movement and improper loading of the weight-bearing surfaces in the joint. Additionally, strengthening optimizes normal alignment of the bones to slide on each other as they were meant to. Finally, exercise in general moves joints, stimulates receptors, manages localized swelling, and promotes a healthy joint—and thus reduces pain.

The stronger a person is, the better stability they have from the foot through the spine. This contributes immensely to balance. Also, strength and power allow a person to catch himself/herself effectively after losing their balance. Numbers of falls can be prevented, resulting in a decline in hip fractures, concussions and more serious head injuries, and broken arms.

There is a direct correlation with strength, function, and life longevity. In general, the stronger a person is, the healthier they are and the more likely they will live a long and functional life.

BENEFITS OF EXERCISE

Exercise reduces negative stress and improves sleep, appetite, lean body mass, bone density, heart efficiency, blood sugar metabolism, hormonal production and management, and cognition.

Exercise stokes the furnace. Regular activity causes your body to burn more energy. Strength training builds lean muscle mass. This muscle mass is "metabolically active," meaning that it burns calories just by existing. The more you have, the more you burn.

Suggestions for a well-rounded program include balance exercise, flexibility training through stretching, resistance training for strengthening, cardiovascular training through walking/jogging/running, and a cool down for recovery and safety. Competitive sports for the older adult are essential in adding a sense of purpose. They are highly social and motivating.

OTHER ASPECTS OF HEALTH

DIET

Diet is important for recovery and maximizing response to the activities above. The scope of this manual is not to provide specific advice on diet. I encourage you to read additional resources provided at the end of this book if you would like more specific information. However, I can safely suggest that your diet should consist of whole foods (vegetables, lean meats, nuts, and fruits), minimal breads, as little refined sugar as possible, minimal refined processed foods (such as chips, crackers, and snack foods), minimal alcohol, and plenty of plain water.

HYDRATION

Regarding water, hydration is very important as you age. It improves the function of cells (specifically muscle and brain cells) so they can operate maximally. Dehydration can cause a number of issues, including fatigue, dizziness, irritability, tissue injury, constipation, and urinary tract issues, to name a few. Making sure you are getting enough water throughout the day will help your body function optimally. And as mentioned immediately above, drink plenty of "plain water." Avoid high sugar and caffeinated beverages as sources of hydration. If you spend time in hot weather, an occasional sports drink is alright. Cut your sports drink with water to dilute it, while getting more water into your system.

REST

Sleep is essential for the body to repair daily wear and tear. Avoid exercising late at night (right before bedtime) as it can affect sleep quality and the ability to fall asleep. Establish a regular time to go to bed.

Recommendations are to get seven to nine hours of sleep nightly, leaning toward the longer duration. Chronic sleep deprivation has been linked to shorter lifespan.

Many people believe hours before midnight count more than after. Sleep in a room as quiet and dark as possible, using a sleep mask and ear plugs if needed. Avoid alcohol and caffeine before bed, as they disrupt sleep cycles and do not allow for deep, restful sleep to occur. Make sure there is a bedside lamp accessible at night if you need to use the bathroom. Take extra care when walking at night in the dark, as the risk of falling increases substantially.

MINDFULNESS

Finally, I would like to discuss the topic of mindfulness. Mindfulness, as I consider it, is the ability to look into your life and how you feel about yourself and your surroundings. This is most generally done through quiet, intentional resting and meditation.

I have always considered meditation a necessary component to overall health and wellness. However, I virtually never made time for it because I was usually too busy trying to be the best at whatever I was doing at that time. It wasn't until after I became ill and was searching for answers and solutions that I came full circle to this area of practice. I had tried everything to recover and heal, and in those moments when I felt well, I would return to my previous driven, high stress, and anxious lifestyle, only to have my symptoms reoccur.

It wasn't until I serendipitously met with an old friend, who had experienced a very similar condition, that I was truly introduced to the practice of being mindful through meditation. Needless to say, I take time every single day, frequently multiple opportunities, to reflect on the moment, embrace it, and find gratitude for where I am now. I routinely practice every morning, sitting quietly, setting my intentions (what I want for myself and my feelings and emotions) for the day and my life, return to that practice early afternoon to re-ground myself, and finally end my day with gratitude that I have the opportunity to be part of this life and all of its wonderful offerings, big and small.

Meditation and mindfulness have a depth of benefits that have been shown over history. Studies continue to show evidence that meditation and mindfulness practices have a place in future medicine, health, and wellness. I can truly say that it saved me from my ego and gave me the beneficial opportunity to appreciate and love myself for who I am, deepening my commitment to myself, family, friends, and society. Without it, I would have remained a ship lost at sea, looking for any horizon to sail to.

There are many options for incorporating meditation in some form into your life, and I strongly encourage everyone to find a practice that fits them. There are a number of coaches, books, magazine resources, and smartphone apps that I am grateful to know of and will recommend in the resources section of this book. Please consider making this an active part of your daily practice. In my heart, I do know you will find great benefit from incorporating this essential practice into your life.

BRAIN HEALTH

One thing that many people don't take into consideration is the substantial control you have over your brain health and cognition. In many instances, it isn't until people notice the subtle and insidious signs of cognitive decline that they take stock in keeping their wits sharp and honed.

To note, cardiovascular exercise is a great way to help improve brain health. Increased exercise in this form results in an increase in blood flow to the brain as well as other tissues. Additionally, the demand in the body and brain for more oxygen-rich blood results in an adaptive response. The body continues to develop a greater concentration of small tributaries of blood flow, known as capillary beds. Over time, these adaptations help provide healthy blood flow to all tissues in the body, and especially the brain.

Cognitive challenges help areas of the brain remain functioning at their highest level of ability. In many cases, these challenges can cause an improvement in function, including memory and processing speed. I encourage you to explore the large variety of brain training programs available today. Puzzles and games, when challenging and rewarding, are great ways to promote cognitive function. I caution you to find a program, especially if you are paying a fee for access, that is supported by research and evidence. Review the program thoroughly before committing financially.

When evaluating clients, one question I ask is, "What are your hobbies?" and furthermore, "Do you have any active hobbies?" It is not surprising to find clients spend most of their time engaged in what I call "passive hobbies," such as watching television, reading, crocheting, and doing crossword puzzles. Though there are many passive hobbies that can be beneficial for mental function, it is essential that you have an active hobby, such as walking, resistance training, hiking, cycling, swimming, or an organized activity such as yoga, group exercise classes, martial arts, or the like. Find an active hobby that you are engaged in, inspired by, and motivated to make part of your life. Not only can you meet new people but also challenge your body and brain to practice something new, improving brain function and general health.

Finally, I want to provide a comment on being uncomfortable. Not in the sense of having pain or discomfort, but in the idea of challenging yourself with new things. Pick up an instrument, learn a language, take the long way home, hike on variable terrain (i.e., hillsides, grassy surfaces, uneven ground) and in different directions, like backward and sideways. These little challenges will not only improve your general function but keep your brain flexible and nimble.

CHAPTER 11

Putting It All Together

Get a journal, a small notebook, or whatever you can to log your benchmarks and activity sessions. Think of this as your Mobility Training Program. For technologically savvy persons, there are smart phone apps that allow you to track your progress with regularly performed routines. This can be very helpful, as you are then able to organize and track the amount of activity you complete and your progress in specific benchmarks.

Here's an idea for journaling your activities or benchmarks:

» On the first page of your journal, write down five goals for your Mobility Training Program. Maybe a goal is to get off the floor or be able to get up from a chair easier. Set a goal for whatever you choose as important and use the information in this book to problem-solve improving it.

» Create a chapter for each area of focus discussed in this manual. For example, chapter 1 should be *Posture*. Perform the posture benchmark. If it is easy, write down on the first page "Date – Easy." If the next time it is difficult, write down on the next line "Date – Difficult," then document what activity you did to improve, such as, "Spent 10 minutes at the wall working on holding a tennis ball in place behind my head."

WHAT ARE APPROPRIATE GOALS?

Many people identify an area they are good at and set goals in this area. We have a tendency to steer away from our deficiencies and focus on areas where we excel.

Direct your focus to areas of deficiency. It is important to recognize your weak points and work to build them up to match your strengths. If reaching overhead is a benchmark you struggle with, focus your energy on improving this area. If posture is optimal, table the exercise until the next round of benchmark assessments. If balance is lacking, which certainly can be true for anyone, depending on how advanced the tests are, spend some time in this area. Whatever your goal is overall, make sure you are improving your deficiencies along with your strengths to develop a solid foundation of skill. All of the recommended tasks above complement each other in maximizing mobility.

Below is a sample table to use to track your status with each activity.

Date:

Activity	Status (Met, Not Met)	Response
Posture		
Lying On Your Stomach		
Getting Off the Floor		
The Squat		
Overhead Reach		
Plank Position		
Single-Limb Stance		
60 Second Sit-Stand Test		
Endurance Test		

Use the table above as a checklist to review weekly or monthly. As you move through the items, rate each of them with a pencil. *Met* means you are easily able to complete the required benchmark. *Not Met* means that either the benchmark is difficult or you are unable to complete it in its entirety. The response column allows you to write a plan, whether it is for goal setting or documenting your progress with a routine. Use a pencil so you can update the table. If this sample table does not work for you, build your own tracking system. The most important thing is to track your performance regularly, at least every month.

RECOMMENDED PRESCRIPTION

Of the nine benchmarks above, if you struggle to complete all of them, you have some work to do to recover your abilities. If you only struggle with three, then you're doing pretty well.

Dedicate 30 minutes on as many days of the week as possible to the process. It is my belief that *everyone* is capable of dedicating 20-30 minutes daily to improving their wellness and maximizing their function. Those who are not able to make the time are dedicating time and resources to other things—be it work, volunteerism, or other hobbies. It boils down to *priorities.*

My clients are routinely caregivers to family members and friends as well. I coach many of them in the perspective that if you are unable to take care of yourself, how can you take care of others or maximize the joy you get from your personal endeavors and hobbies? Pain and weakness can be a drain on inspiration. Resolving those issues will spill over into great rewards in the rest of your life's works.

So—back to keeping it simple: dedicate 20-30 minutes daily to three or four of the benchmarks you struggle with. Be sure to get four to five days of practice in each week. Spend 10 minutes per benchmark.

As your benchmark is met, table it and focus on other areas.

As described early on in this book, if you find you are not deficient in any benchmarks, you're in a great place and should move to the maintenance phase. Recheck your benchmarks regularly (every 15-30 days) to ensure you are not falling behind in any areas.

THE MAINTENANCE PHASE

If your benchmark assessment checks out, the important thing is to remain as active as possible. Find "active hobbies" that you enjoy and spend time doing them. It is important to have at least one "active hobby" that you engage in daily. These include gardening and yard work, golfing, fitness/wellness, hiking, cycling, running, yoga, tennis, or other sporting activities, etc. Having an active hobby will keep you moving in the maintenance phase and help you keep up on your benchmarks and maximize your mobility. They also help you enjoy your life!

CHAPTER 12

Motivation/Inspiration

An administrator of an assisted living facility mentioned that "clients do very well when participating in formal therapy. However, when they are transitioned to either an independent exercise program or even a small group, many lose the inspiration they once had to work toward continual improvement. How can we keep people motivated to continue their program of personal development?"

This is also my greatest challenge, as a clinician working with persons with neurological conditions. The gains frequently are small, steady, and slow. Because of this, people often lose sight of the goals they have established. They progressively perform their home program less frequently, until finally it collects dust on the nightstand or worse, disappears into the void of paperwork from the hospital.

I don't blame them for not adhering to the program. I think it's safe to say most people have difficulty maintaining regular physical activity for one reason or another. Many of us have work, family, and life obligations that consume our time and energy, leaving little to no resources left for routine exercise. I'm as guilty of it as my clients are. I go stretches of time, short and long, in which I'm unable to achieve my daily goals for exercise. This leaves me frustrated and concerned with my ability to commit to my personal health and also to other commitments such as my family, clients, and coworkers.

HOW TO STICK TO YOUR EXERCISE PROGRAM

Don't feel alone if sticking with your program is something you struggle with. Following are some suggestions and strategies to help you stick to a routine of regular physical activity:

» Foremost, *set goals*. Set weekly goals that allow you to measure your success. Choose goals that are absolutely measurable and easily analyzed. For example, set goals for how often you are going to practice. The recommendations I provide are a good place to start.

  a. Daily practice is ideal but not always realistic in your life. Maybe you're a person who is more comfortable with a goal of something like this: "Four days per week, I will spend 30 minutes working on my areas of improvement."

  b. Consider weekends as bonus days to get in your frequency of practice. If you have busy weekdays, it is frequently easier to set aside 30 minutes on Saturday and Sunday mornings for a routine like this. It also takes the pressure off of getting in your routine on weekdays and makes it more realistic to stick to the program.

» If you do not achieve your weekly goal, *do not get discouraged.* Consider why you didn't meet your expectations and make realistic changes to improve your success.

» *Journal your routines.* Use an app on your smartphone to track your daily workouts, not only to compare to previous performances, but also as inspiration for your dedication to your routine. Since I started using this method in 2012, I have currently logged over 400 workouts. That means over the past three years, I have chosen to take time out of my schedule to exercise approximately every three days. Some weeks, I was able to achieve five days per week (which I am personally proud of), while in others it was one to two days per week (which I consider an area needing improvement). But overall, every three days is a meaningful dedication to my physical development and something I am willing to boast about!

» *Write down your goals.* As previously suggested, keeping a journal of your progress is paramount in maintaining forward momentum. Make the first page of your journal a list of your goals. Goals can be as fundamental as, "I will be able to get out of bed efficiently in the morning." Goals can also relate to your roles or hobbies, such as "I will be able to consistently garden this season."

We as therapists use models to identify areas of deficiency in our clients, and then use these same models to establish goals across spectrums of "Classification of Function." The World Health Organization has a model titled the "International Classification of Functioning, Disability, and Health," or the ICF model. It looks at aspects of an individual's abilities across a number of domains. The three domains are *Body Structure and Function, Activity,* and *Participation.*

An example of using this model to recognize and set goals is as follows: An individual has difficulty with posture and overhead reach (Body Structure and Function), making it difficult to swing their arms efficiently and effectively or walk sufficient distances (Activity), which prevents them from golfing nine holes with friends or family (Participation).

We clinicians are skilled in using this model to recognize relationships between each area, but you don't have to link each domain to effectively set goals with each. Think of your life as a flow between each domain. The suggestions in this book are more classified in the domains of Body Structure and Function, as well as Activity. Use this as a guide to set goals in these areas.

Recognize what is important to you in the Participation domain, such as playing a round of golf, carrying a grandchild, hiking on a trail, mountain biking your favorite route, hunting upland birds or big game, working in your woodshop, or spending time in your garden. Jot down meaningful goals in your journal that you can reflect on daily to see if you are progressing toward them.

This leads me to the next suggestion for motivation:

» *Reflection.* No program is effective without time spent reflecting on your progress toward your goals. Set aside 15-20 minutes weekly or a couple times per week to look at your goals and see if you are moving toward them. For each goal, make a mental or physical note as to how you are getting closer to achieving it. What is preventing you from making progress? What barriers exist that you can easily knock down to finally meet the goal for this week? If you set a goal of performing this program four days per week but only found you had time on Monday and Thursday to squeeze it into the busy schedule, can you commit 30 minutes Saturday and Sunday morning to meet the goal?

» *Make it social.* As I commented on above, there is strength in numbers. Rally family members and friends to join you in the program. I find nothing more effective at keeping me participating regularly in my program than the camaraderie of friends and my wife. Make it a family plan, where grandparents exercise with grandchildren. Small group exercise is a powerful tool and can be utilized in any household or center. There should be lots of discussion about purpose and open dialogue between people as to what helps them achieve success with these activities or any other exercise program they choose to engage in.

If you find it difficult to recognize factors that contribute to your motivation, my final recommendation is to seek out professionals skilled in helping people recognize ways to inspire you to commit to your goals. Physical therapists, personal trainers, and wellness coaches all have the knowledge and tools to help you identify what works for you as an individual. Don't give up because you feel adrift. Look for a beacon to bring you in to shore and get you grounded in your personal development.

CONCLUSION

I believe that as a person ages, he/she develops wisdom and maturity that can only come over time. It is a tragic ending to a beautiful story when grandparents and parents are reduced to requiring help with basic daily activities, not because of disease or illness, but because they have lost the capability gradually through a lack of activity. I am humble yet proud to offer and suggest that the information contained in these pages can help make a difference in the quality of life a person experiences as they age—that they can maintain a more independent lifestyle with these simple steps.

What I offer is empowerment: Recognize that you have regenerative abilities at any age and you can reverse or prevent a decline in your physical abilities.

In the rehabilitation setting, I have worked with individuals with a variety of diagnoses, from stroke to spinal cord injury, from Parkinson's disease to West Nile viral encephalopathy, from joint replacement to failure to thrive. I have observed and assisted these individuals in an effort to improve their independence, basic mobility skills, and quality of life.

THE IMPORTANCE OF CONTINUED MOVEMENT

It wasn't until recently that I realized something: All people have the capacity to carry out movements that allow them to function maximally in their daily lives. If they do not perform these movements on a regular basis, they will lose the ability to do so. As the old adage states, "A rolling stone gathers no moss."

As you age, your abilities are not governed by the aging process entirely, but by your willingness to maintain your capacity to carry out the movements required in your daily life.

Observe children. They're fascinating when you look at the amount of energy they have, and the awkward postures they are able to get into. As I watch my 18-month-old daughter, she bends, twists, and rests in a deep squat position. Whether she is focused on constructing something or recovering from her older sister's roughhousing, she moves in ways that I find natural and innate. And the energy. Oh my! Anyone who has children is aware of this. Kids have abundant and instantly accessed energy that allows them to cause mass chaos in a short period of time. It has been said that the average toddler covers 47 football fields in one day!

I believe that a proactive approach to assisting older adults in this country would significantly reduce the number of people who end up in a nursing home, unable to care for themselves and too much of a burden on their families to allow them to stay at home. Helping them maintain or regain their physical abilities so they can keep living an independent life would be a win for them, their families, and the healthcare system. People don't realize how much capability they are losing through inactivity until they are injured or their abilities decline past the point of no return.

This book is not intended to be a textbook on my philosophy, values, and beliefs about how to sidestep the aging process. It is a manual that suggests some basic exercise movements that can be used to achieve and maintain what I call *benchmarks for functional capacity.* The information is concise and easy to understand.

My goal for this manual is to be read in one week and applied immediately.

This book offers the aging population what I feel is an essential tool-kit of activities to maximize their mobility. These activities maintain and improve not only strength, but also joint health and range of motion, functional capacity of the muscle and body as a whole, and ongoing independence with participation in life's greatest roles.

I want every adult over the age of 50 to realize that more greatness is yet to come. With proper maintenance and care, the body has no reason to decline so rapidly. With a little attention and investment, you can get better, stronger, and more capable. You can continue hiking in the foothills, golfing 18 holes, carrying and playing with your grandchildren, or just about any idea you have for yourself.

My own health issues have given me a different perspective on the limitations a diagnosis can impose—or not, if you choose to reject the standard projected outlook. I have seen people exceed those expectations because they chose not to accept them.

For centuries, other societies have demonstrated not only longevity but also robust functional capacity into old age. One of those attributes is the constant movement they engage in that is required for normal daily activities in their culture.

Recently, I was on a quest for self-improvement. I was trying to find a direction that inspired me to take action. My profession allows me to spend a specific amount of time with each individual person, addressing their needs and providing a plan of attack to recover independence and quality of life. But I wanted to do more than that.

I have set a goal of helping more than one person at a time—I wanted to help a large number of people effectively and efficiently. I feel that with this short manual, I have accomplished that.

Even if, right now, you pass all the benchmarks with flying colors, this manual gives you the tools you need to continue moving and maintaining your physical capabilities well into old age. Commit to continued movement and working to improve your strength and abilities, and you will have the tools necessary to live an independent and functional life. Much of your destiny is in your hands. With the right maintenance process, you will be able to live life to the fullest.

AFTERWORD

As described in my note at the beginning of this book, the goal of this manual is to reach as many people as possible with this information. I can only reach one person at a time in my clinical practice. It's exciting to think of the possibility of hundreds or even thousands of people reading this manual and putting the core concepts to work in their lives on a daily basis. What's even more exciting is believing that people have the desire to do this *before* they develop severe limitations that are difficult to recover from. My vision is to maximize prevention as much as it is to recover lost function.

Group exercise programs are fantastic, though they have their limitations. They are not individualized enough, and the activities may not be scaled down to meet the needs of each specific person in the class.

I have been amazed over the years as I observe many people with conditions that have sidelined them. A large number of those same people have recovered function that has allowed them to return to their roles. I would be naïve to suggest that we can outlast time and cheat aging, but I can say that people's capacity to remain and become more mobile, strong, agile, flexible, and independent is limited only by their dedication to improving these aspects of their lives.

Individualized instruction, whether it be a personal trainer, fitness professional or physical therapist, is still that: Individualized and "one person at a time." That's an impossible way to impact society. Hopefully, this information can broaden who I touch, and encourage us all to take control of our abilities to maximize our mobility in the years ahead.

RESOURCES

I've included a list of resources for a deeper dive into specific areas of health and wellness. I encourage you to eagerly seek out and review these resources, take pieces and insights you feel add value to your quest, and don't worry about what doesn't fit your goals. Revisit the concepts and expand by finding other resources on similar topics.

The Longevity Diet – by Dr. Valter Longo (*The Longevity Diet: Discover the New Science Behind Stem Cell Activation and Regeneration to Slow Aging, Fight Disease, and Optimize Weight.* Avery, 2018)

» According to Dr. Longo, through what foods we consume and when we consume them, we can dramatically affect the various processes occurring in our bodies to promote health, healing, and longevity.

The Blue Zones – by Dan Buettner (*The Blue Zones: Lessons for Living Longer From the People Who've Lived the Longest.* National Geographic, 2010)

» Dan Buettner sought to determine the characteristics of long-lived societies around the world and shares common beliefs about longevity and happiness.

Healthy at 100 – by John Robbins (*Healthy at 100: The Scientifically Proven Secrets of the World's Healthiest and Longest-Lived Peoples.* Ballantine Books, 2007)

» Another book that explores the habits of unique societies with increased "health spans."

Soft-Wired – by Michael Merzenich (*Soft-Wired: How the New Science of Brain Plasticity Can Change Your Life,* 2nd edition. Parnassus Publishing, 2013)

» Dr. Merzenich explores and presents the evidence showing us that at any age, we can positively impact our cognitive function and the resulting abilities, as well as wellness and happiness, with strategic activities and games to promote strengthening the connections in our brains.

Institute of Functional Medicine – https://ifm.org

» This developing field of medical practice explores the role and relationship the environment plays in our health and illness, including from diet, allergies, toxins, and stress. Certified clinicians provide thorough assessments and examinations, as well as education.

These resources are not the "end all, be all" of information. This single page of resources doesn't begin to scratch the surface, but they are a starting point to inspire you that at any age, in any condition, a positive course of action has the ability to yield results to shift the direction you're traveling. It's never too late.

ACKNOWLEDGMENTS

I would like to start by thanking my family and especially my wife, Katie, for her support and encouragement throughout this project— for letting me have the many mornings I rose well before sunrise with a pot of coffee to pour my thoughts and ideas into this. The quiet time to focus on what I felt was necessary to share was well supported. I love you all more than you'll ever know.

Thank you to my parents, Myron and Cheryl, for supporting me and teaching me to have the will and desire to pursue my dreams and to foster and nurture my growth as a human being and physical therapist. You taught me passion and purpose in life. I will always remember this, and I cherish and love you for it.

Over the years, I have had many colleagues and peers come and go. I want to thank all of them for their contributions in shaping my vision of what it means to be a care provider. I would like to include Char Roy and Renee Hawkins, two of the most compassionate and skilled clinicians I've had the opportunity to learn from. The most influential ones helped elevate the bar of helping others reach their goals, however lofty those goals may have been or will be. Never stop striving for a better world.

The people who helped review this document in its early stages have truly contributed and helped carry this project to its final stage.

From patients (privacy protected, but you know who you are) and family members to peers (Christine Walsh and Dr. Rodde Cox), my coach Tanya Penny (a truly gifted spiritual guide to growth and healing), and mentors (Dr. Vic Kadyan, Dave Fleckenstein, Shelley Thomas, and John Amtmann), without your words of encouragement and emotional backing (not only on this project, but also personally and professionally), I would not have realized what a diamond in the rough this was. You absolutely provided me with the courage and passion to believe in what I want to share and contribute to all people looking for a better and more satisfying life.

Finally, to my consulting team at Aloha Publishing in Eagle, Idaho: I cannot be more grateful. From the first day, you supported and encouraged me with suggestions and ideas on how best to get my point across and develop my message. You reinforced for me that this was a worthwhile endeavor.

ABOUT THE AUTHOR

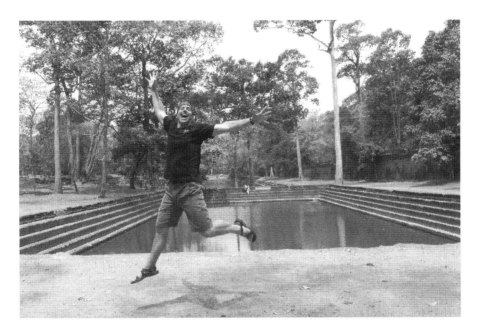

Joseph Wegley is a licensed physical therapist in Boise, Idaho, with 15 years of experience in the area of adult neurological rehabilitation. He is currently a clinical coordinator of adult neurological rehabilitation at St. Luke's Rehabilitation Hospital, where he has contributed to the development and refinement of directed programs.

Joe is board certified in Neurological Physical Therapy with the American Board of Physical Therapy Specialties. He also is recognized as a Certified Exercise Physiologist with the American College of Sports Medicine, as well as a Certified Brain Injury Specialist with the Brain Injury Association of America.

Joe began his pursuit toward the profession of physical therapy by working as a physical therapy aide at an outpatient clinic within a nursing home environment. It was here that he first helped aging adults achieve improved function through exercise and activity and was inspired to continue in the field.

Joe volunteers and contributes to the board of directors for the local nonprofit, LIMBitless. This organization's mission is to help persons with mobility limitations to achieve their goals through community engagement and through recreation and a vision of inclusion. The LIMBitless Challenge, an annual event, consists of teams of volunteers and participants (individuals with mobility limitations, either walking or wheelchair propelled) supporting each other on a 1.6-mile climb on the primitive hiking trail of Table Rock in Boise, Idaho.

His greatest vision is to see everyone share something with another being, a gift they can give to another to help elevate them. If we all made the effort to give some time, wisdom, knowledge, or support to one other person, imagine the positive change we could make in this world and the potential rippling effect it would make over time. Just one person . . .

Joe attended Montana Tech in Butte, Montana, where he achieved a Bachelor of Science degree in occupational safety and health with an emphasis on applied health sciences in 2001. He graduated from the University of Montana in Missoula, Montana, with a clinical Doctorate in Physical Therapy in 2004. His first position was as a staff physical therapist at Elks Rehabilitation Hospital in Boise, Idaho.

A portion of the profits from this book will be donated to a local nonprofit supporting children and aging adults to improve their opportunities and quality of life.

Made in the USA
Las Vegas, NV
17 April 2023

70689458R00068